Nomad - Rusty cells

Toxic Metal Detox

Nomad – Rusty Cell

Toxic Metal Detox

Copyright © *Levitas One*, 2024

All Rights Reserved

What are the NoMAD Plans?

Developed by Dr Ash Kapoor, the NoMAD Plans represent a transformative approach to health and wellness that combines the wisdom of ancestral practices with contemporary medical insights. The name "NoMAD" not only suggests a journey through the intricate realm of health but also stands for its foundational principles: Nutritional Optimisation, Mindful Adaptation, and Detoxification.

At the heart of NoMAD is the 6R Framework—Restore, Release, Repair, Renew, Reframe, and Represent. This methodology addresses the root causes of illness, combats chronic inflammation, and cultivates authentic vitality, guiding individuals through a transformative process.

Tailored specifically to each individual, NoMAD journeys are meticulously crafted to rebalance the body, strengthen the mind, and rejuvenate overall health. By integrating ancestral practices with cutting-edge, innovative treatments—all under strict medical oversight—NoMAD Plans offer a personalised pathway to sustainable, long-lasting well-being that resonates with your unique life circumstances.

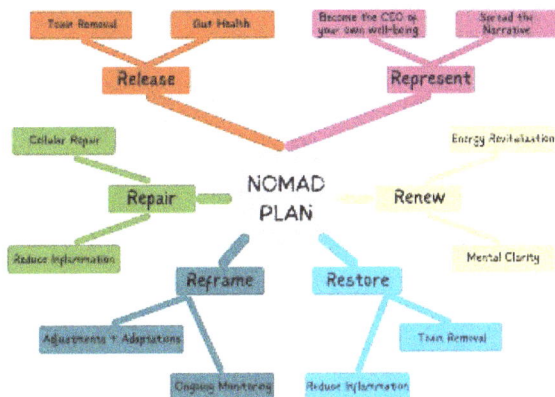

Levitas One:
"As Is In, As Is Out"

Reflecting the belief that our internal well-being is mirrored in our external environment. Founded by Dr Ash Kapoor, Levitas One serves as the vehicle for delivering NoMAD's treatment plans. It envisions a healthcare future where patients are at the centre of a fully integrated, multidisciplinary approach. Guided by Nomads 6 Rs—Restore, Release, Repair, Renew, Reframe, and Represent—Levitas One empowers self-care through personalised guidance and minimal intervention, promoting long-term health, balance, and sustainability.

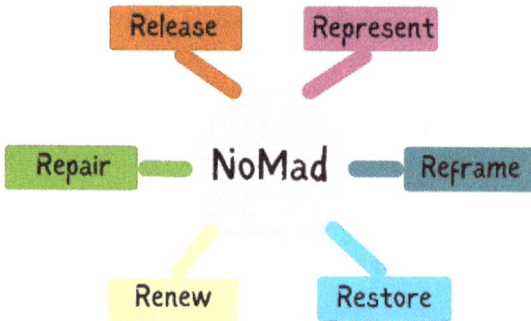

Contents

Preface ix

Chapter 1: Understanding Heavy Metals 1
Definition and Classification 1
Case History: 1
Historical Context and Usage...3

Chapter 2: Pathways of Absorption 7
How Heavy Metals Enter the Body 7
Factors Influencing Absorption Rates 9
Summary...12

Chapter 3: The Ubiquity of Heavy Metals 13
Industrial Revolution and the Surge of Heavy Metals in the
Environment...13
Comparisons of Metal Exposure: Ancient Times vs. Modern Era 14
Occupational Exposure in Different Eras..15
Summary...17

Chapter 4: Heavy Metals in Ancient Civilisations 19
Use in Medicine, Cosmetics, and Technology 19
Health Impacts: Ancient Records and Modern Interpretations.............21
Summary...23

Chapter 5: The 19th and Early 20th Century 25
The Industrial Revolution and Urbanisation 25
Case Studies: Lead Paint, Mercury in Medicine.......................................26
Summary...29

Chapter 6: The Mid-20th Century to Present Day 31
Environmental Policies and Awareness (1940s–1960s) 31
Case Studies: Minamata Disease and Leaded Gasoline...........................32
The Rise of Heavy Metal Contamination in the Post-Industrial World34
Summary...35

Chapter 7: Mechanisms of Toxicity 37
Cellular and Molecular Effects of Heavy Metals......................................37
Chronic vs. Acute Exposure..40
Summary...42

Chapter 8: Systemic Health Impacts of Heavy Metals 44
Neurological Damage...44

Cardiovascular and Renal Issues 46
Impacts on Reproductive Health 47
Summary 49

Chapter 9: The Silent Epidemic – Why Heavy Metal Toxicity Is Often Missed 51
Why Heavy Metal Toxicity Is Often Missed 51
Challenges in Diagnosis 53
Summary 55

Chapter 10: Traditional Diagnostic Methods 57
Blood and Plasma Testing 57
Urine and Hair Analysis 59
Summary 61

Chapter 11: Advanced Diagnostic Techniques 63
Oligoscan: Pros and Cons 63
Emerging Technologies in Metal Detection 65
Summary 67

Chapter 12: Case Studies in Diagnosis 70
Misdiagnosed Cases and Lessons Learned 70
Diagnostic Challenges Across Eras 73
Summary 75

Chapter 13: Medical Interventions for Heavy Metal Toxicity 77
Chelation Therapy: Mechanisms, Risks, and Benefits 77
Other Pharmaceutical Interventions 80
Combining Medical Interventions with Functional Approaches 81
Summary 82

Chapter 14: Functional Medicine and Alternative Therapies for Heavy Metal Detoxification 84
Nutritional Support and Detox Protocols 84
Herbal Remedies and Natural Chelators 86
Integrative and Holistic Therapies 88
Summary 90

Chapter 15: Intravenous Therapies for Heavy Metal Detoxification 92
Overview of Drip Therapies: Vitamin C, Glutathione, EDTA 92
Efficacy and Safety Concerns 95
Case Histories of IV Therapy Success 96
Summary 98

Chapter 16: General Treatment Protocols for Heavy Metal Detoxification 100
Combining Medical and Functional Approaches 100

Tailoring Treatment to Individual Cases 103
Case Histories of Customised Detox Protocols 104
Summary..106

Chapter 17: Case Histories of Heavy Metal Toxicity Across Different Eras 108
Early 20th Century: Occupational Exposure and Industrialisation 108
Mid-20th Century: Environmental Contaminations and Public Health Disasters 110
21st Century: Chronic Low-Level Exposure and Modern Health Impacts 113
Summary..114

Chapter 18: Global Distribution of Heavy Metals and Environmental Justice 116
Geographic Variations in Heavy Metal Exposure..................................116
Impact of Industrialisation in Developing Countries 118
Environmental Justice and Policy Implications.....................................120
Summary..122

Chapter 19: Heavy Metals in Dentistry – A Hidden Health Risk...124
The Use of Heavy Metals in Dental Practices 124
Health Risks and Controversies...126
Emerging Alternatives and Safe Practices 128
Summary..130

Chapter 20: Policy and Advocacy – Addressing Heavy Metal Exposure Through Environmental Regulations and Public Health Initiatives 132
Environmental Regulations Across the Eras 132
The Role of Public Health Advocacy in Shaping Policy 135
Challenges in Policy Implementation and Enforcement.......................136
Summary..138

Chapter 21: The Future of Heavy Metal Exposure – Emerging Contaminants, Technological Advancements, and New Frontiers in Detoxification 140
Emerging Contaminants and New Sources of Heavy Metal Exposure 140
Technological Advancements in Monitoring and Mitigation 142
Future Directions in Heavy Metal Research and Policy.......................145
Summary..147

Chapter 22: Final Thoughts and Call to Action – Creating a Safer Future 149
Summary of Key Points 149

Recommendations for Future Research, Policy, and Clinical Practice150
Call to Action: Moving Toward a Healthier Future.................................153
Conclusion 154

Glossary **156**
References **162**

Preface

My name is Dr Ash Kapoor, and I have spent nearly 35 years practising medicine, dedicating my career to understanding the complexities of human health. Throughout this journey, I have been deeply affected by the widespread ignorance surrounding the impact of heavy metal toxicity. Heavy metals, with their long biological half-lives—often extending beyond 30 years—can accumulate in the body over time, leading to profound and often insidious health consequences.

As a clinician, I've observed first-hand how this silent form of toxicity manifests in my patients. For over a decade, I have conducted extensive testing and assessments, and the results have been alarming: no one is immune to the effects of heavy metals. Whether it's lead, mercury, cadmium, or arsenic, these toxic elements infiltrate our systems through a multitude of sources—food, water, air, and even everyday household items. Before the 1980s, lead was the primary culprit, contributing to widespread health issues. Today, we face an increasing burden of aluminium, mercury, and other emerging contaminants. Despite the growing body of research highlighting the dangers of these metals, mainstream medicine often overlooks or underestimates their role in chronic disease.

This book aims to bridge that knowledge gap and provide a comprehensive overview of heavy metal toxicity, its history, health impacts, and treatment strategies. It is designed not only for healthcare professionals but for anyone seeking to understand how these hidden toxins may be affecting their health and well-being. By shedding light on the science and evidence behind heavy metal exposure, my hope is to empower individuals with the knowledge they need to take proactive steps toward protecting their health.

We cannot afford to continue masking symptoms with pharmaceutical solutions while ignoring the root causes of illness. Instead, we must strive to uncover the true sources of disease and address them with evidence-based, patient-centred approaches. I believe that the more we understand about heavy metal toxicity, the better equipped we will be to make informed decisions that benefit both our health and the health of future generations.

This book is my contribution to that mission. I invite you to join me in this exploration of the silent intruders—heavy metals—and discover what we can do to mitigate their effects and move toward a healthier, more informed future.

Dr Ash Kapoor

Chapter 1: Understanding Heavy Metals

Definition and Classification

Heavy metals are a group of metals and metalloids that have relatively high density and atomic weight. Although the term "heavy metals" is often associated with toxicity, it actually refers to a wide range of elements, some of which are essential for life. Broadly, heavy metals can be classified into **toxic heavy metals** and **essential heavy metals**.

- **Toxic Heavy Metals** include elements like lead, mercury, cadmium, and arsenic. These metals have no known beneficial role in the human body, and even at low exposure levels, they can disrupt biological systems, causing severe health problems.
- **Essential Heavy Metals**, such as zinc, copper, and iron, are required in small amounts for various biochemical processes. These elements are often described as **"keys"** that unlock critical biological functions. For example, zinc is necessary for immune function, and iron is vital for oxygen transport in the blood.

However, even essential heavy metals can become toxic when present in excess. It's a delicate balance — like a "double-edged sword." Just as keys open doors, too many or misplaced keys can cause damage. On the other hand, toxic heavy metals behave like **"rogue agents"**, invading and disrupting essential cellular processes, much like intruders in a secure system. Once in the body, they can interfere with enzymes, damage DNA, and lead to systemic health issues, from neurological damage to organ failure.

Case History:

The Romans, unknowingly, used lead for their plumbing systems, pipes, and water vessels. Lead is malleable and easy to work with, which made it ideal for constructing their elaborate aqueduct systems. However, this decision had serious consequences. Lead from the pipes leached into the water supply, slowly poisoning the population. Some historians believe that this widespread lead poisoning may have contributed to the decline of the Roman Empire. Symptoms of lead toxicity — such as cognitive impairment, infertility, and gout — were reported in ancient Roman texts, though the cause wasn't understood until centuries later.

Common Heavy Metals: Lead, Mercury, Cadmium, Arsenic, etc.

Heavy metals vary in toxicity and how they affect the body. Here are some of the most well-known toxic heavy metals:

1. **Lead**

    Lead is one of the most pervasive environmental toxins. Once absorbed, it accumulates in the bones and soft tissues, particularly the brain and kidneys. It interferes with the formation of haemoglobin, which is critical for oxygen transport, and damages the nervous system. Chronic lead exposure can cause cognitive decline, developmental delays in children, and even death in cases of acute poisoning.

    Analogy: Lead acts like a "thief" in the bloodstream, displacing essential minerals like calcium and iron, and weakening bones and organs.

2. **Mercury**

    Mercury is unique in that it can exist in multiple forms — elemental, inorganic, and organic (such as methylmercury, found in fish). Each form has different toxic effects. Methylmercury, for example, is a potent neurotoxin that crosses the blood-brain barrier and damages neurons. Long-term mercury exposure can result in tremors, memory loss, and, in extreme cases, irreversible brain damage.

Case Study: In the Minamata disaster in Japan, industrial mercury waste contaminated the water, and over decades, people consuming fish from the bay developed severe neurological impairments.

3. Cadmium

Cadmium exposure comes mainly from industrial processes and cigarette smoke. It accumulates in the kidneys, leading to renal dysfunction and bone demineralisation, causing diseases like osteoporosis.

Analogy: Cadmium is like a "silent invader" in the kidneys, slowly degrading their filtering abilities without causing immediate symptoms.

4. Arsenic

Arsenic, found in contaminated groundwater in various parts of the world, is highly carcinogenic. Chronic arsenic exposure leads to skin lesions, cancer, and cardiovascular diseases.

Case Study: In Bangladesh, millions of people have been exposed to arsenic-contaminated drinking water, leading to what the World Health Organisation calls "the largest mass poisoning of a population in history."

These metals are commonly found in a variety of everyday sources. Lead is found in old paint, batteries, and plumbing. Mercury accumulates in seafood like tuna and swordfish. Cadmium is used in batteries and is found in cigarette smoke, while arsenic is present in contaminated water and certain foods like rice. Understanding the sources of these metals is crucial for both preventing exposure and recognising the subtle signs of poisoning.

Historical Context and Usage

Throughout history, humans have used heavy metals in medicine, industry, and everyday life, often with dangerous consequences.

Heavy metals have been both a boon and a curse. While their properties made them useful in construction, medicine, and art, their toxicity was often overlooked until it was too late.

- **Medicine:**

In ancient China, mercury was used as part of elixirs meant to grant immortality. Emperor Qin Shi Huang, who unified China, was one of the most famous victims of mercury poisoning. Believing that the elixirs would extend his life, he unknowingly consumed mercury regularly, which eventually led to his death.

Similarly, in the 18th and 19th centuries, mercury was a common treatment for syphilis in Europe. Although it had limited efficacy, the side effects, including severe mouth ulcers, kidney failure, and neurological issues, were devastating.

Case Study: Famous explorer Lewis of Lewis and Clark suffered from mercury poisoning during his journey, as the explorers carried mercury-laden pills with them as medicine.

- **Cosmetics and Art:**

Lead-based makeup was used by both the Ancient Egyptians and Greeks. Cleopatra is said to have used lead-based kohl to line her eyes, which may have contributed to lead poisoning. Similarly, the Victorians and Renaissance artists used lead-based paints and powders, which caused long-term health issues.

Case History: Renaissance painter Caravaggio was known for his use of vivid colours in his paintings, many of which contained lead-based pigments. It's speculated that his later-life violent outbursts and erratic behaviour were linked to lead poisoning, a common affliction of artists at the time.

- **Industry:**

With the advent of the Industrial Revolution, the use of heavy metals surged, particularly in manufacturing, plumbing, and machinery. Lead was widely used in construction materials, pipes, and even gasoline. Mercury was used in hat-making, giving rise to the term **"mad as a hatter"** due to the neurological damage it caused in workers exposed to mercury fumes.

Case Study: In the 19th century, hat makers in Europe and the United States commonly suffered from mercury poisoning due to the use of mercuric nitrate in the felting process, leading to tremors, irritability, and cognitive impairment. This condition became so prevalent that it gave birth to the "Mad Hatter" character in Lewis Carroll's *Alice in Wonderland*.

The widespread and unregulated use of heavy metals throughout history has left a lasting legacy on human health. Ancient civilisations didn't understand the risks, but modern science has uncovered the dangerous effects these metals have had for centuries. Today, despite regulations and advances in technology, heavy metals continue to pose a global health risk, making it essential to learn from history to prevent future exposures.

Summary: Understanding Heavy Metals

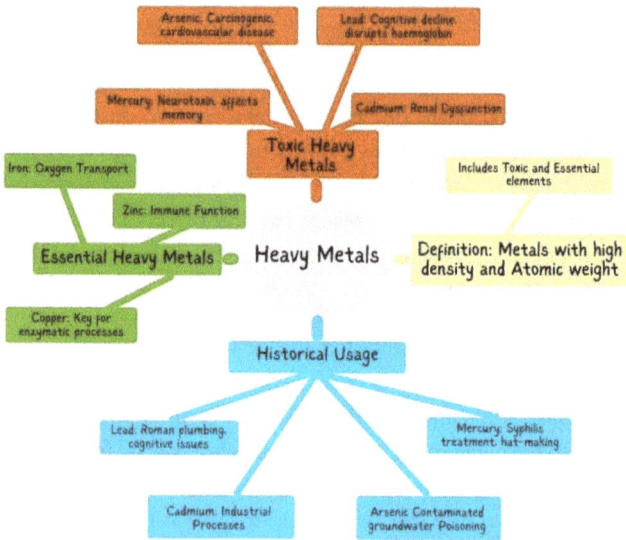

Toxic Heavy Metals
- Arsenic: Carcinogenic, cardiovascular disease
- Lead: Cognitive decline, disrupts haemoglobin
- Mercury: Neurotoxin, affects memory
- Cadmium: Renal Dysfunction

Essential Heavy Metals
- Iron: Oxygen Transport
- Zinc: Immune Function
- Copper: Key for enzymatic processes

Heavy Metals
- Includes Toxic and Essential elements
- Definition: Metals with high density and Atomic weight

Historical Usage
- Lead: Roman plumbing, cognitive issues
- Cadmium: Industrial Processes
- Arsenic: Contaminated groundwater Poisoning
- Mercury: Syphilis treatment, hat-making

Chapter 2: Pathways of Absorption

How Heavy Metals Enter the Body

Heavy metals can enter the body through various routes: ingestion, inhalation, and dermal absorption. Each of these pathways allows toxic metals to bypass the body's natural defences and infiltrate vital organs and tissues. To conceptualise this, imagine heavy metals as **"invisible invaders"** entering through multiple gates and dispersing silently throughout the body.

- **Ingestion**
  Ingestion is one of the most common ways heavy metals enter the body. Contaminated food, water, and soil are typical sources. Once ingested, heavy metals like lead, arsenic, and mercury pass through the digestive system, where they can be absorbed into the bloodstream. For instance, methylmercury in fish, arsenic in groundwater, and lead in contaminated food products pose serious health risks.

  Analogy: Ingestion acts as a wide-open gate. If the gatekeepers (our food and water) are contaminated, heavy metals can easily find their way inside, like unwanted guests entering a house.

  Case History: Mercury from Seafood

  A 45-year-old woman who regularly consumed tuna and swordfish began to experience fatigue, memory loss, and difficulty with fine motor skills. Medical tests revealed elevated mercury levels. The source was traced to her diet, which included fish known to accumulate high levels of mercury. This case illustrates how a common dietary habit can result in chronic heavy metal exposure, leading to neurological impairment.

- **Inhalation**
  Heavy metals such as lead, mercury, and cadmium can also enter the body through inhalation. This is particularly dangerous for people working in industries such as mining, welding, and battery manufacturing, where metal dust and fumes are present. Once inhaled, metal particles can bypass the body's respiratory defences, settling in the lungs and being absorbed into the bloodstream.
  Analogy: Inhalation is like leaving the backdoor open for intruders. Metal particles slip in unnoticed with every breath, especially in occupational settings.

Case Study: Cadmium Exposure in Factory Workers

A group of workers in a battery factory, exposed to cadmium dust daily despite using basic protective equipment, developed kidney damage over time. They were inhaling cadmium particles that settled in the respiratory tract and eventually entered their bloodstream. Years later, many of these workers experienced chronic kidney disease, highlighting the long-term risks of inhaling heavy metal particles.

- **Dermal Absorption**
  Dermal absorption, or the entry of metals through the skin, is less common but still significant, particularly for metals like arsenic, chromium, and nickel. This can occur when individuals handle contaminated materials without protection or come into contact with polluted soil or water. The metals penetrate the skin's outer layers and eventually enter the bloodstream.
  Analogy: Dermal absorption is like an invisible hand reaching through the skin's barrier, slowly introducing metals into the body. Though not as immediate as ingestion or inhalation, it is still a notable pathway for exposure.

Case Study: Arsenic in Contaminated Groundwater

A farming community in Bangladesh faced chronic exposure to arsenic due to contaminated groundwater. The residents not only ingested arsenic but also experienced dermal exposure as they used the water for bathing and irrigation. Over time, residents developed characteristic skin lesions and other arsenic-related health issues, highlighting how dermal exposure, combined with ingestion, can exacerbate health outcomes.

Factors Influencing Absorption Rates

The rate at which heavy metals are absorbed into the body varies significantly depending on several factors, including **age**, **nutritional status**, **overall health**, and the **type and duration of exposure**. Understanding these factors helps explain why certain individuals are more susceptible to heavy metal toxicity than others. A helpful analogy is to think of the body as a **"sponge soaking in toxic water"** — the degree of absorption depends on how porous the sponge is and the type of water it encounters.

- **Age**
  Age is a critical determinant of absorption. Children, for instance, are more vulnerable to heavy metal poisoning because their bodies are still developing and their metabolic systems are more efficient at absorbing nutrients — and toxins. For example, children absorb approximately 50% of the lead they ingest, compared to only 10% in adults. This increased absorption rate, combined with developing organs, makes children particularly susceptible to neurological damage from heavy metal exposure.
- **Analogy:** Imagine a young, porous sponge soaking up more water compared to an older, less absorbent sponge. Children's bodies, like the young sponge, absorb more heavy metals and hold onto them longer.

Case Study: Lead Exposure in Children

A 6-year-old boy living in a house with peeling lead-based paint developed severe behavioural issues and learning difficulties. His parents, unaware of the lead hazard, did not suspect poisoning until tests revealed alarmingly high levels of lead in his blood. This case underscores how age-related factors make children especially vulnerable to absorbing and retaining heavy metals.

- **Nutritional Status**
  Nutritional deficiencies can also increase the body's absorption of heavy metals. When the body is deficient in essential minerals like calcium, iron, or zinc, it becomes more likely to absorb toxic metals, which can mimic these nutrients and take their place in the body's biochemical processes. For example, when calcium is lacking, lead can replace calcium in bones, leading to greater accumulation and toxicity. Similarly, iron deficiency can increase cadmium and lead absorption, worsening their toxic effects.

  Analogy: A depleted sponge will absorb more water than one that is already saturated. Likewise, a nutrient-deficient body is more likely to "soak up" heavy metals, exacerbating the effects of exposure.

Case Study: Iron Deficiency and Cadmium Exposure

A 35-year-old woman working in a factory with cadmium exposure suffered from iron deficiency. Over time, cadmium accumulated in her kidneys, causing significant damage. Her nutritional deficiency made her body more susceptible to absorbing cadmium, demonstrating the critical link between nutritional status and heavy metal absorption.

- **Overall Health**
  Health conditions such as compromised liver or kidney function can significantly impact the body's ability to process and eliminate heavy metals. Individuals with kidney or liver disease are less capable of excreting toxins, leading to higher retention and greater health risks. Additionally, autoimmune diseases or chronic illnesses can make individuals more vulnerable to the toxic effects of heavy metals.

Analogy: A damaged or compromised sponge will not only absorb more toxic water but also struggle to release it, holding onto the poison longer than a healthy sponge.

Case Study: Mercury Retention in Individuals with Kidney Disease

A 60-year-old man with chronic kidney disease consumed fish high in mercury. Because his kidneys could not filter toxins effectively, mercury accumulated in his body, leading to worsening kidney function and neurological symptoms. This case shows how pre-existing health conditions can exacerbate heavy metal toxicity.

- **Type and Duration of Exposure**
  The form of heavy metal and the duration of exposure also influence absorption rates. Organic mercury (methylmercury), found in seafood, is more readily absorbed than inorganic mercury, making dietary sources of mercury particularly dangerous. Acute exposure to high levels of lead can cause immediate symptoms, while chronic, low-level exposure may take years to manifest noticeable health effects.
  Analogy: A sponge can absorb water quickly or slowly, depending on the amount and duration of exposure. Similarly, the body's interaction with heavy metals depends on whether it is faced with a single large dose or small amounts over a prolonged period.

Case Study: Chronic Arsenic Exposure from Contaminated Water

Residents of a small town in South America drank arsenic-contaminated water for decades. Although the concentration of arsenic was not immediately lethal, chronic exposure resulted in long-term health issues, including skin cancer and cardiovascular diseases. This case illustrates how prolonged, low-level exposure can lead to severe health outcomes, even when symptoms are not initially apparent.

Summary

This chapter details how heavy metals enter the body and the various factors that influence their absorption, using case histories and analogies to provide a deeper understanding of the topic. These insights lay the groundwork for understanding how heavy metals impact health and why exposure can vary significantly between individuals.

Summary: Pathways of Absorption

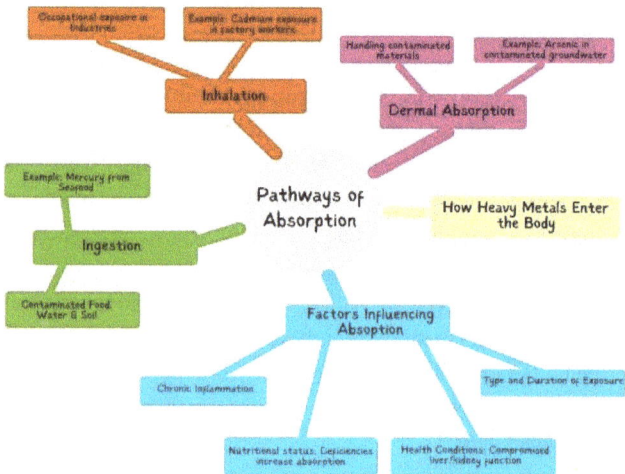

Chapter 3: The Ubiquity of Heavy Metals

Industrial Revolution and the Surge of Heavy Metals in the Environment

The Industrial Revolution, beginning in the late 18th century, marked a turning point in the widespread presence of heavy metals in the environment. As industrial activities expanded rapidly, heavy metals such as lead, mercury, and cadmium were released into the air, soil, and water in unprecedented quantities. This era, often seen as a symbol of human progress, also sowed the seeds of a silent environmental disaster. Heavy metals were incorporated into various products, including paints, plumbing materials, machinery, and batteries, making them omnipresent in the Industrialised world.

During this period, the use of heavy metals grew exponentially as they were valued for their versatility, conductivity, and resistance to corrosion. Factories spewed pollutants into the air, while industrial waste was discharged into rivers and lakes, contaminating water supplies. For example, lead was used extensively in pipes and construction, while mercury was essential for manufacturing processes like felt production in the hat industry.

Analogy: Imagine the world during the Industrial Revolution as a "toxic cauldron," with factories acting as enormous chimneys releasing invisible toxic fumes. These fumes settled on crops, penetrated water bodies, and seeped into the very fabric of society. Heavy metals were like "ghosts" that haunted industrial landscapes, invisible yet deeply destructive.

- **Case Study: Cadmium in Industrial Waste and Community Health**
A small industrial town in England became a hub for metal refining in the early 19th century. Factories producing batteries and pigments released significant amounts of cadmium into the

local environment. Decades later, residents began to experience a mysterious rise in kidney disease and bone disorders. An investigation revealed that the soil, water, and even local crops were heavily contaminated with cadmium, which had accumulated in the community's food chain over the years. This case exemplifies how industrial waste can have long-lasting impacts on community health.

- **Environmental Fallout**
  The impact of heavy metals from the Industrial Revolution lingers to this day. Lead contamination in soil remains a significant issue in urban areas where old buildings with lead-based paints were constructed. Similarly, mercury persists in waterways, accumulating in fish and posing a health risk to consumers. It is estimated that nearly 20 million children in developing countries are exposed to lead contamination from industrial sources such as smelting plants and battery recycling facilities.

The environmental consequences of the Industrial Revolution serve as a stark reminder that the use of heavy metals, while beneficial in the short term, has serious long-term repercussions for human health and the environment.

Comparisons of Metal Exposure: Ancient Times vs. Modern Era

The presence of heavy metals in human society is not new. Throughout history, humans have been exposed to heavy metals, though the sources and extent of exposure have changed dramatically over time. While ancient civilisations like the Romans and Egyptians encountered heavy metals in limited contexts — primarily through the use of metals in cosmetics, medicine, and rudimentary plumbing — the scope of exposure in modern times is far more pervasive and dangerous.

In ancient times, exposure was typically localised and affected specific groups such as artisans, alchemists, and miners. For example,

Roman plumbers and water engineers frequently worked with lead pipes, which exposed them to lead dust and fumes. However, these exposures were limited to specific trades, and the general population was less affected.

In contrast, the modern era has seen a dramatic increase in widespread exposure due to industrial activities, technological advancements, and the use of heavy metals in consumer products. Today, the general population is exposed to a variety of heavy metals through air pollution, contaminated food and water, household products, and even electronic devices.

Analogy: Think of ancient exposure as a "local infection" that affected specific parts of society, whereas modern exposure is like a "systemic disease" that impacts the entire body of society. Heavy metals have permeated every corner of modern life, from our homes to our workplaces and even the natural environment.

Case Study: Lead in Ancient vs. Modern Times

In ancient Rome, lead pipes used for plumbing were the primary source of lead exposure. Only those who were directly involved in construction or had prolonged contact with water from these pipes experienced significant poisoning. In contrast, modern exposure to lead is far more widespread. Leaded gasoline, widely used in the mid-20th century, dispersed lead into the atmosphere, affecting millions of people globally. Even though leaded gasoline has been phased out, residual contamination in soil and dust continues to pose a risk, particularly in urban environments.

The comparison between ancient and modern exposure illustrates how technological advances, while beneficial in many ways, have also introduced new and pervasive risks that were previously unimaginable.

Occupational Exposure in Different Eras

Occupational exposure to heavy metals has evolved significantly over the centuries, reflecting changes in industry, technology, and safety regulations. In ancient times, miners, metalworkers, and alchemists were at the highest risk of heavy metal exposure. Miners working in Greek and Roman mines often inhaled metal dust and fumes, leading to respiratory illnesses and early death. Metalworkers, particularly those involved in smelting and alloying metals, were exposed to high levels of lead and mercury, resulting in neurological and cognitive issues.

With the onset of the Industrial Revolution, new occupations emerged that involved direct contact with heavy metals. Factory workers in industries like battery manufacturing, paint production, and chemical processing were frequently exposed to lead, mercury, cadmium, and chromium. Safety standards were minimal, and personal protective equipment (PPE) was rare. Many workers suffered from chronic illnesses, often without knowing the cause.

In the 20th century, occupational safety standards began to improve, particularly after the establishment of organisations like OSHA (Occupational Safety and Health Administration) in the United States. Even so, occupational exposure remains a significant concern in certain industries. Workers in electronics recycling, welding, and smelting are still at high risk of exposure, particularly in countries where safety regulations are not strictly enforced.

Analogy: Occupational exposure can be likened to "walking on a tightrope" — workers balance the benefits of employment with the risks of toxic exposure. Without proper safety measures, one misstep can lead to severe health consequences.

Case History: Lead Exposure in Battery Factory Workers (1950s)

In the 1950s, a battery factory in the United States became notorious for lead poisoning among its workers. Employees handled lead plates and compounds daily without proper ventilation or protective gear. Over time, workers developed symptoms such as anaemia, abdominal pain, and cognitive decline. It wasn't until multiple workers died that the factory was shut down, and the issue of occupational lead exposure gained national attention.

This case, and many others like it, underscores the importance of implementing stringent safety standards to protect workers from the harmful effects of heavy metal exposure.

Summary

Chapter 3 explores how the Industrial Revolution exponentially increased the presence of heavy metals in the environment, creating a long-lasting legacy of contamination. It compares exposure levels between ancient times and the modern era, showing how technological advances have both alleviated and exacerbated the risks. Furthermore, it examines occupational exposure across different eras, highlighting the evolution of safety standards and ongoing challenges.

With detailed case studies and analogies, this chapter emphasises the pervasive and persistent nature of heavy metal exposure and its impact on human health. It sets the stage for understanding the health implications of heavy metals, which will be explored in the following chapters.

Summary: The Ubiquity of Heavy Metals

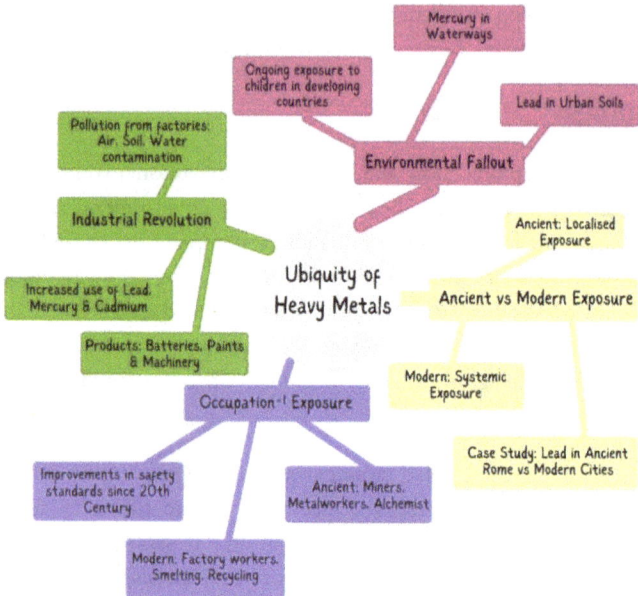

- Mercury in Waterways
- Ongoing exposure to children in developing countries
- Lead in Urban Soils
- Environmental Fallout
- Pollution from factories: Air, Soil, Water contamination
- Industrial Revolution
- Ancient: Localised Exposure
- Increased use of Lead, Mercury & Cadmium
- Ancient vs Modern Exposure
- Ubiquity of Heavy Metals
- Products: Batteries, Paints & Machinery
- Modern: Systemic Exposure
- Occupational Exposure
- Case Study: Lead in Ancient Rome vs Modern Cities
- Improvements in safety standards since 20th Century
- Ancient: Miners, Metalworkers, Alchemist
- Modern: Factory workers, Smelting, Recycling

Chapter 4: Heavy Metals in Ancient Civilisations

Use in Medicine, Cosmetics, and Technology

Heavy metals were widely used in ancient civilisations, valued for their unique properties and believed to possess medicinal and mystical qualities. However, their use often came at a high cost, as societies unknowingly exposed themselves to the toxic effects of these substances. Understanding the historical use of heavy metals helps contextualise their longstanding impact on human health and culture.

1. **Medicine**

   In ancient times, metals such as mercury, lead, and arsenic were incorporated into various medicinal preparations. These metals were believed to have therapeutic properties, capable of curing illnesses or even extending life. Mercury was commonly used in Traditional Chinese Medicine as an ingredient in elixirs meant to grant immortality. Unfortunately, its toxic effects often led to severe health problems and even death.

   Analogy: Mercury in ancient medicine was like a "double-edged sword" — while it was thought to have life-extending properties, it often delivered a fatal blow due to its toxicity.

   Case History: The Death of Emperor Qin Shi Huang

   Emperor Qin Shi Huang, the first emperor of unified China, was obsessed with achieving immortality. His alchemists prepared elixirs containing mercury, which he consumed regularly. Instead of gaining eternal life, he suffered from severe mercury poisoning, resulting in tremors, mental decline, and ultimately, death. This case exemplifies how the lack of scientific understanding in ancient times led to fatal outcomes from heavy metal use.

2. **Cosmetics and Personal Care**
   Ancient Egyptians, Greeks, and Romans used lead and mercury in cosmetics. Egyptian women applied lead-based kohl to their eyes to create dark eyeliner, a fashion statement that persisted for centuries. Lead was also used in skin creams and powders to whiten the complexion, a practice that continued into the 18th century in Europe.
   Analogy: The use of heavy metals in cosmetics was like "putting beauty before health" — while enhancing appearance, these products slowly poisoned their users.

Case Study: Cleopatra's Use of Lead-Based Cosmetics

Cleopatra, the famous Egyptian queen, was known for her striking beauty and heavy use of cosmetics. She applied lead-based eye makeup daily, unaware of its toxic effects. While there is no direct evidence that this contributed to her demise, many women of her time suffered from skin lesions, neurological symptoms, and infertility due to chronic lead exposure.

3. **Technology and Daily Use**
   Ancient civilisations used heavy metals in a variety of technologies. The Romans constructed aqueducts with lead pipes, the Greeks used copper alloys for tools and weapons, and the Chinese used mercury in tombs as a means of preserving artefacts. While these applications showcased the versatility and utility of heavy metals, they also introduced significant health risks.
   Analogy: Heavy metals in ancient technology were like "hidden dangers" — useful tools that came with an unseen cost to health.

Case History: Lead Poisoning in Roman Plumbing

The Roman Empire's advanced plumbing system was one of its great engineering achievements. Lead pipes supplied water to homes, bathhouses, and public fountains. However, the widespread use of lead led to chronic poisoning among the population. Symptoms such as gout, infertility, and mental decline were prevalent among the Roman elite, who had greater access to piped water. While the exact role of lead poisoning in the decline of the Roman Empire is debated, it is clear that its health effects were significant.

Health Impacts: Ancient Records and Modern Interpretations

Historical records provide fascinating insights into the health impacts of heavy metals on ancient populations. Ancient texts from civilisations such as Egypt, Greece, and Rome describe symptoms of heavy metal poisoning, though they lacked the knowledge to identify these substances as the cause. Modern scientific research has allowed us to reinterpret these historical accounts, providing a clearer picture of the toxic legacy of heavy metal use.

1. **Ancient Egypt**
   Egyptian medical texts, such as the Ebers Papyrus (circa 1550 BC), mention symptoms that align with heavy metal poisoning, including "burning of the skin," "mental confusion," and "paralysis of the limbs." The papyrus describes treatments that likely worsened the condition, as many included the use of additional metals like copper and arsenic.

   Modern Interpretation: Historians believe that many of these symptoms were due to lead and arsenic poisoning from cosmetics, pottery, and medical concoctions. For example, symptoms of anaemia and fatigue were likely caused by lead exposure from everyday household items.

   Case History: Anaemia in the Pharaoh's Court

   The mummified remains of Egyptian royalty have shown high levels of lead and arsenic, indicating chronic exposure. Analysis of these remains revealed signs of anaemia and osteoporosis, common symptoms of heavy metal toxicity. This evidence suggests that even the elite, who had access to the best medical care, suffered from the adverse effects of heavy metals.

2. **Ancient Greece and Rome**
   Greek physicians like Hippocrates and Roman writers like Pliny the Elder described conditions that we now know were likely caused by heavy metal poisoning. Pliny noted that miners often succumbed to a mysterious disease characterised by coughing, shortness of breath, and early death — symptoms that align with lead and mercury poisoning. Similarly, Hippocrates wrote about "colic" and other gastrointestinal issues affecting metalworkers.
   Modern Interpretation: Many of these ailments were likely caused by inhalation of metal fumes and ingestion of contaminated water. These records provide a glimpse into the occupational hazards faced by ancient metalworkers.

   Case Study: Greek and Roman Miners

   Greek and Roman miners often worked in confined spaces with poor ventilation, exposing them to high levels of metal dust and fumes. Analysis of skeletal remains from ancient mining sites shows signs of chronic respiratory disease and bone damage consistent with lead and mercury exposure.

3. **Ancient China**
   Alchemists in ancient China believed mercury and arsenic had life-extending properties and used them in various medicinal elixirs. Historical records describe symptoms such as trembling hands, confusion, and hallucinations among alchemists and emperors who consumed these elixirs.
   Modern Interpretation: These symptoms were likely due to mercury and arsenic poisoning. The deaths of several Chinese emperors have been attributed to their consumption of these toxic substances in pursuit of immortality.

   Case History: The Toxic Quest for Immortality

   Emperor Jiajing of the Ming Dynasty (1507–1567) was obsessed with prolonging his life through the use of "immortality pills" containing mercury and arsenic. He suffered from severe tremors, memory loss, and paranoia, all symptoms of heavy metal poisoning. His death is believed to have been caused by his toxic obsession with immortality.

Summary

Chapter 4 delves into the historical use of heavy metals in medicine, cosmetics, and technology, highlighting how these substances, while revered for their unique properties, often caused significant harm. Through detailed case histories and modern scientific interpretations, this chapter provides a comprehensive look at how ancient societies suffered from heavy metal exposure without understanding its dangers. From Cleopatra's use of lead-based makeup to Emperor Qin Shi Huang's fatal consumption of mercury, these stories serve as powerful reminders of the lasting impact of heavy metals on human health and history.

This chapter sets the stage for understanding how the lessons from ancient civilisations can inform modern approaches to managing heavy metal exposure and toxicity. It transitions seamlessly into the next chapters, where the focus will shift to how heavy metal use surged during the Industrial Revolution and how modern society continues to grapple with the consequences.

Summary: Heavy Metals in Ancient Civilisations

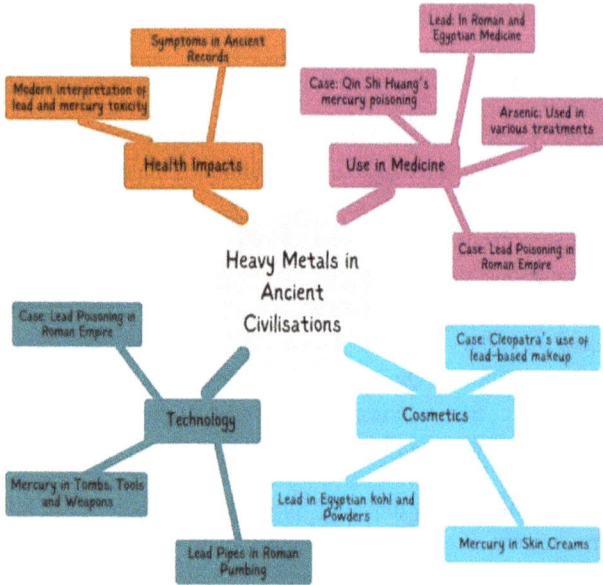

Heavy Metals in Ancient Civilisations

Health Impacts
- Symptoms in Ancient Records
- Modern interpretation of lead and mercury toxicity

Use in Medicine
- Lead: In Roman and Egyptian Medicine
- Case: Qin Shi Huang's mercury poisoning
- Arsenic: Used in various treatments
- Case: Lead Poisoning in Roman Empire

Technology
- Case: Lead Poisoning in Roman Empire
- Mercury in Tombs, Tools and Weapons
- Lead Pipes in Roman Plumbing

Cosmetics
- Case: Cleopatra's use of lead-based makeup
- Lead in Egyptian kohl and Powders
- Mercury in Skin Creams

Chapter 5: The 19th and Early 20th Century

The Industrial Revolution and Urbanisation

The 19th century marked a period of dramatic transformation as Industrialisation and urbanisation reshaped societies across the globe. The advent of machinery and mass production brought about unprecedented growth in industries such as mining, metallurgy, and manufacturing. However, this industrial boom also led to a significant rise in heavy metal contamination. As factories proliferated and cities expanded, the environment became increasingly saturated with toxic metals like lead, mercury, and cadmium.

During the Industrial Revolution, heavy metals were used in a wide variety of applications. Lead was a key component in plumbing, paints, and gasoline additives. Mercury was used in thermometers, dental amalgams, and the manufacture of felt hats. Cadmium was employed in battery production and pigment manufacturing. These metals, valued for their durability, conductivity, and other properties, were essential for the burgeoning industrial economy.

Urbanisation further compounded the problem as people flocked to cities in search of work. The rapid expansion of cities meant that homes, factories, and industrial plants were often built side by side. This proximity led to increased exposure to airborne heavy metal particles and contaminated water sources. Cities became hotspots of pollution, with factories releasing metal-laden smoke into the air and waste into rivers.

Analogy: Imagine the rapidly growing cities of the 19th century as **"smoke-filled cauldrons"**, where toxic fumes from factories mixed with household pollutants to create a toxic stew. The people living in these urban centres, particularly the working class, were like "ingredients" simmering in this cauldron, absorbing toxic metals with each breath they took and every sip of water they drank.

Case Study: Lead Poisoning in Victorian England

In Victorian England, lead poisoning became a widespread issue, particularly among children. Many urban homes used lead pipes for water supply, and lead-based paints were ubiquitous in households. Children, who are naturally more prone to hand-to-mouth behaviour, often ingested lead dust from peeling paint and contaminated soil. By the late 19th century, the health effects of lead poisoning—such as cognitive impairment, developmental delays, and physical weakness—were well-documented, yet few regulations were in place to limit exposure.

The environmental and health impacts of the Industrial Revolution were profound, with heavy metals seeping into nearly every aspect of urban life. As cities grew and industrial activities increased, so did the public health crisis caused by heavy metal contamination.

Case Studies: Lead Paint, Mercury in Medicine

The widespread use of lead in paint and mercury in medicine during the 19th and early 20th centuries led to numerous public health tragedies. Despite early recognition of their toxic effects, heavy metals continued to be used due to a lack of understanding and regulation.

1. **Lead Paint: A Silent Danger in Homes**
   Lead-based paint was popular in the 19th century because it was durable, water-resistant, and had a bright finish. It was used extensively in both residential and public buildings, making it a pervasive source of lead exposure, particularly for children. **Analogy:** Lead paint in homes was like a **"time bomb on the walls"**—an ever-present danger that slowly poisoned families over time. When the paint began to chip and peel, lead dust was

released into the environment, contaminating floors, toys, and even food.

Case History: The Tragedy of Lead Paint Exposure

One notorious case in early 20th-century Boston involved a group of children living in an apartment complex painted with lead-based paint. Over the course of a few years, these children developed a range of symptoms, including severe anaemia, abdominal pain, and learning disabilities. Medical professionals, unfamiliar with the signs of lead poisoning, initially misdiagnosed the children with various other conditions. It wasn't until one child experienced seizures and died that an autopsy revealed high levels of lead in his body. The subsequent investigation uncovered dangerously high levels of lead in the paint throughout the building. This tragic incident prompted one of the first major public health investigations into the dangers of lead-based paint, though it took several more decades for comprehensive regulations to be enacted.

2. **Mercury in Medicine: A Misguided Cure**
   In the 19th century, mercury was widely used in medicine to treat conditions like syphilis, a sexually transmitted infection that was rampant at the time. Known as **"quicksilver"**, mercury was believed to purge the body of illness through its purgative and laxative effects. However, mercury is highly toxic, and its use often resulted in more harm than good.
   Analogy: Mercury in medicine was like **"a wolf in sheep's clothing"**—a substance that appeared to cure, yet wreaked havoc on the body, causing symptoms that could mimic or even worsen the original illness.

Case History: Mercury Poisoning in Syphilis Patients

The famous composer Ludwig van Beethoven is thought to have suffered from mercury poisoning due to treatments he received for syphilis. Throughout his life, Beethoven experienced symptoms such as mood swings, abdominal pain, and memory loss—classic signs of mercury toxicity. His autopsy revealed significant damage to his liver and kidneys, organs commonly affected by mercury poisoning. Though mercury was eventually replaced by safer treatments, its use in medicine led to countless cases of poisoning, adding to the burden of illness rather than alleviating it.

3. **"Mad Hatter" Syndrome: Occupational Mercury Exposure**

The term **"mad as a hatter"** originated from the widespread use of mercury nitrate in the hat-making industry. Hatters who worked with felt soaked in mercury solutions developed symptoms such as tremors, mood swings, and hallucinations.

Analogy:

Mercury exposure for hatters was like **"a slow descent into madness"**—workers inhaled mercury fumes daily, accumulating toxic levels over time, which led to neurological impairment.

Case History: The Hatter's Plight in 19th-Century England

In 19th-century England, hat makers, known as hatters, were exposed to mercury nitrate during the felting process. Prolonged exposure led to a condition known as **"hatter's shakes,"** characterised by uncontrollable tremors. Many hatters also suffered from psychological symptoms, including depression and anxiety, eventually becoming unfit for work. Despite these symptoms being widely recognised, the connection to mercury was not understood until the early 20th century, by which time countless workers had suffered irreversible damage.

These case studies highlight the pervasive and insidious nature of heavy metal exposure during the 19th and early 20th centuries. Whether through lead paint in homes or mercury in medical treatments, the widespread use of these metals caused untold harm to human health, laying the foundation for future regulations and safer practices.

Summary

Chapter 5 examines how the industrial and medical uses of heavy metals during the 19th and early 20th centuries led to widespread public health crises. The Industrial Revolution and subsequent urbanisation turned cities into hotspots of contamination, while the unregulated use of lead and mercury in consumer products and medicine resulted in numerous cases of poisoning and long-term health issues.

Through detailed case histories and vivid analogies, this chapter illustrates how heavy metals like lead and mercury, once considered essential for industrial and medical progress, became silent killers that ravaged communities. The lessons learned from these tragic experiences paved the way for the eventual recognition of heavy metals' toxic effects and the development of regulations aimed at protecting public health.

The stage is now set to explore how environmental policies and public awareness began to address these issues in the mid-20th century, as discussed in Chapter 6.

Summary: The 19th and Early 20th Century

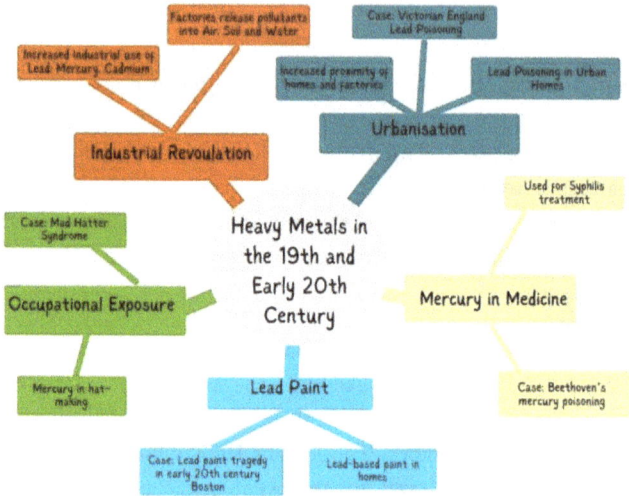

Factories release pollutants into Air, Soil and Water

Case: Victorian England Lead Poisoning

Increased Industrial use of Lead: Mercury, Cadmium

Increased proximity of homes and factories

Lead Poisoning in Urban Homes

Urbanisation

Industrial Revoulation

Used for Syphilis treatment

Case: Mad Hatter Syndrome

Heavy Metals in the 19th and Early 20th Century

Occupational Exposure

Mercury in Medicine

Mercury in hat-making

Lead Paint

Case: Beethoven's mercury poisoning

Case: Lead paint tragedy in early 20th century Boston

Lead-based paint in homes

Chapter 6: The Mid-20th Century to Present Day

Environmental Policies and Awareness (1940s–1960s)

The mid-20th century marked a turning point in the way society viewed and managed heavy metal contamination. During the 1940s and 1950s, industrial activities were at an all-time high, and environmental pollution became increasingly visible. Rivers turned colours from industrial discharge, air quality declined, and communities experienced severe health problems. However, it wasn't until the 1960s that public awareness and scientific research began to uncover the long-term health impacts of heavy metals on humans and the environment.

The rise of environmental awareness can be traced back to key events and influential figures such as Rachel Carson, whose ground-breaking book *Silent Spring* (1962) exposed the dangers of pesticides and other pollutants. While Carson's work primarily focused on chemical pesticides, it sparked a broader environmental movement that also targeted heavy metal pollution. As people became more conscious of environmental issues, advocacy for cleaner air, water, and soil grew stronger.

Analogy: Environmental pollution during this era was like **"a rising tide of toxins"** that slowly flooded the ecosystem. Communities living near factories and industrial sites were like residents stranded in a toxic flood, their health and well-being gradually eroded by invisible contaminants.

In response to public pressure, governments began to establish environmental regulations. In the United States, the Clean Air Act (1963) and the Clean Water Act (1972) set the groundwork for limiting emissions of hazardous substances, including heavy metals. Similarly, in Europe, initiatives like the European Environmental

Bureau (established in 1974) focused on reducing industrial pollution and protecting public health.

Case Study: The Minamata Disease Outbreak (1950s–1960s)

One of the most notable examples of heavy metal poisoning during this period is the Minamata disease outbreak in Japan. Minamata disease was caused by methylmercury poisoning, which occurred when a chemical factory dumped industrial waste into Minamata Bay. The mercury accumulated in fish and shellfish, which were then consumed by local residents.

The health effects were devastating—residents developed severe neurological symptoms such as tremors, speech difficulties, and cognitive impairments. Many children were born with birth defects, and the disease claimed hundreds of lives. This tragedy prompted widespread outrage and eventually led to stricter regulations on industrial waste disposal.

The Minamata incident, along with similar cases worldwide, highlighted the urgent need for better environmental protections. It served as a wake-up call for governments and industries, leading to the implementation of environmental policies that continue to shape how heavy metals are managed today.

Case Studies: Minamata Disease and Leaded Gasoline

The mid-20th century saw two major health crises that underscored the dangers of heavy metal exposure: the Minamata disease outbreak in Japan and the widespread use of leaded gasoline in vehicles.

1. **Minamata Disease: The Cost of Industrial Negligence**
   The Minamata disease outbreak in Japan is one of the most severe cases of heavy metal poisoning in history. It began in the 1950s when a chemical factory owned by the Chisso Corporation released methylmercury into Minamata Bay. The mercury contaminated the bay's fish and shellfish, which were

a staple food source for local communities. Over the next few decades, thousands of residents exhibited symptoms of mercury poisoning, including numbness, muscle weakness, vision loss, and cognitive decline. Children born to affected mothers experienced severe developmental issues and birth defects. The company initially denied responsibility, and it wasn't until 1968 that the Japanese government officially recognised the cause of Minamata disease as industrial mercury pollution.

Analogy: The Minamata disease was like **"a silent assassin"**—residents unknowingly consumed contaminated fish, and the mercury gradually attacked their nervous systems, leaving a trail of devastation that spanned generations

Case Outcome: Public outcry and legal battles ensued, ultimately resulting in compensation for victims and stricter environmental regulations. The Minamata incident became a catalyst for global environmental advocacy and led to the formation of international conventions aimed at controlling mercury emissions.

2. **Leaded Gasoline: A Global Epidemic of Lead Poisoning**
   In the early 20th century, lead was added to gasoline to improve engine performance. This practice, however, had disastrous consequences. The combustion of leaded gasoline released lead particles into the air, which were inhaled by millions of people. As vehicle use skyrocketed, so did lead levels in the environment. By the 1960s, researchers began to document the severe health effects of lead exposure, particularly in children. Lead interferes with brain development, leading to cognitive impairments, behavioural problems, and reduced IQ. Despite mounting evidence, the powerful lead industry lobbied against the regulation of leaded gasoline, arguing that the benefits outweighed the risks.

Case Study: The Phasing Out of Leaded Gasoline

It wasn't until the 1970s that countries like the United States began phasing out leaded gasoline. In 1975, the U.S. Environmental Protection Agency (EPA) mandated the gradual reduction of lead in gasoline, a move that was met with fierce resistance from industry. However, the results were clear: as leaded gasoline was phased out, blood lead levels in children dropped dramatically, and health outcomes improved.

Analogy: Leaded gasoline was like **"a slow poison"** being pumped into the atmosphere, affecting not just the drivers but entire communities, especially those living near busy roads and highways.

Global Impact: By the early 2000s, leaded gasoline was banned in most countries, significantly reducing global lead exposure. This shift is considered one of the greatest public health victories of the 20th century, saving millions of children from the devastating effects of lead poisoning.

The Rise of Heavy Metal Contamination in the Post-Industrial World

Despite the progress made in reducing heavy metal pollution in the mid-20th century, the post-industrial world faces new challenges. As industrial activities have shifted to developing countries, these regions now bear the brunt of heavy metal contamination. Electronic waste, or e-waste, has emerged as a significant source of heavy metals such as lead, mercury, and cadmium. Discarded electronics are often processed in informal recycling sectors, where workers, including children, are exposed to toxic fumes and dust.

Additionally, heavy metals are now found in unexpected places, such as household items, electronics, and even certain foods and supplements. While regulations have reduced some sources of exposure, globalisation and the rise of new technologies have introduced new pathways for heavy metal contamination.

Case Study: E-Waste in Developing Countries

Countries like Ghana, India, and China have become dumping grounds for electronic waste from developed nations. Workers in these countries dismantle electronics without proper protection, exposing themselves to high levels of toxic metals. Children working in these informal sectors experience developmental issues, respiratory problems, and skin diseases due to prolonged contact with heavy metals.

Analogy: The modern world is like **"a maze of hidden toxins"**—while we've closed some doors to heavy metals, new ones have opened through the rapid advancement of technology and inadequate global waste management practices.

Summary

Chapter 6 examines the evolution of heavy metal contamination and the policies implemented to address it from the mid-20th century to the present day. Key case studies such as the Minamata disease outbreak and the phasing out of leaded gasoline illustrate the devastating impact of industrial pollution and the hard-won victories of environmental advocacy.

While progress has been made in reducing heavy metal exposure through regulations and public awareness, new challenges have emerged in the post-industrial era. The global shift of industrial activities to developing countries and the rise of e-waste have created new avenues for heavy metal contamination, necessitating continued vigilance and international cooperation.

This chapter sets the stage for understanding the health impacts of heavy metals in modern society, which will be explored in the upcoming sections.

Summary: The Mid-20th Century to Present Day

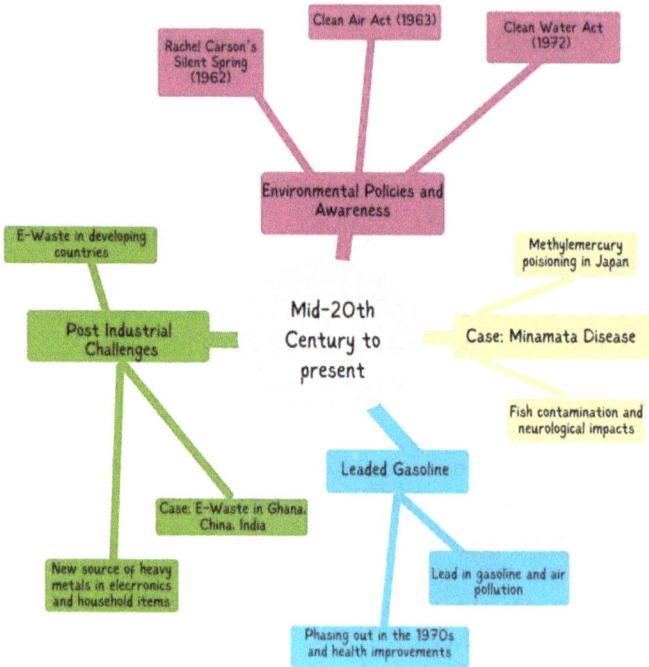

Clean Air Act (1963)

Rachel Carson's Silent Spring (1962)

Clean Water Act (1972)

Environmental Policies and Awareness

E-Waste in developing countries

Post Industrial Challenges

Mid-20th Century to present

Methylemercury poisioning in Japan

Case: Minamata Disease

Fish contamination and neurological impacts

Case: E-Waste in Ghana, China, India

Leaded Gasoline

New source of heavy metals in elecrronics and household items

Lead in gasoline and air pollution

Phasing out in the 1970s and health improvements

Chapter 7: Mechanisms of Toxicity

Cellular and Molecular Effects of Heavy Metals

Heavy metals such as lead, mercury, arsenic, and cadmium are known for their potent toxicity. Once inside the body, these metals disrupt cellular processes at the molecular level, leading to a cascade of health issues. Understanding the cellular and molecular mechanisms of heavy metal toxicity is essential to grasp why these substances are so dangerous, even at low levels of exposure.

1. **Disruption of Enzyme Function**

    Enzymes are proteins that catalyse biochemical reactions, and many rely on essential metal ions (e.g., zinc, copper) to function properly. However, toxic heavy metals such as lead and mercury can displace these essential ions, binding to the enzymes and altering their structure. This disruption can inhibit the enzyme's function, slow down or halt critical biochemical pathways, and produce toxic by-products.

    Analogy: Imagine an enzyme as a "lock" that requires a specific metal ion "key" to open and perform its function. When heavy metals displace the correct ion, it's like trying to unlock a door with the wrong key—the lock becomes jammed, and the door won't open, leading to dysfunction at the cellular level.

    Case Study: Lead and Haemoglobin Synthesis

    Lead interferes with the synthesis of haemoglobin, the protein in red blood cells responsible for oxygen transport. It does so by inhibiting the enzyme **delta-aminolevulinic acid dehydratase (ALAD)**, which is critical in the production of haemoglobin. When lead inhibits ALAD, it causes an accumulation of precursor molecules, leading to anaemia and other blood disorders. This mechanism explains why chronic lead exposure can result in fatigue, pallor, and developmental delays in children.

2. **Oxidative Stress and DNA Damage**
   Heavy metals like arsenic and cadmium are known to induce oxidative stress, a state in which there is an imbalance between the production of free radicals and the body's ability to neutralise them. Free radicals are highly reactive molecules that can damage proteins, lipids, and even DNA. Over time, this oxidative damage can lead to mutations, disrupt cellular signalling, and initiate cancerous processes.
   Analogy: Oxidative stress is like a "fire" that scorches everything in its path, damaging the very building blocks of life. Heavy metals act as "arsonists," sparking these fires by generating excessive free radicals.

Case Study: Arsenic-Induced Oxidative Stress in Cancer Development

Chronic exposure to arsenic has been linked to an increased risk of skin, bladder, and lung cancers. Arsenic generates free radicals that damage DNA, leading to mutations that promote the development of cancer cells. Studies have shown that populations exposed to arsenic-contaminated water have higher rates of these cancers, emphasising the carcinogenic potential of long-term arsenic exposure.

3. **Mitochondrial Dysfunction**
   The mitochondria, known as the "powerhouses" of the cell, generate energy in the form of adenosine triphosphate (ATP). Heavy metals can disrupt mitochondrial function by interfering with the electron transport chain, a series of reactions that produce ATP. Mercury, in particular, is known to bind to mitochondrial enzymes, reducing energy production and causing cell death.
   Analogy: Think of the mitochondria as a "battery" that powers the cell. Heavy metals drain this battery, leaving cells without the energy they need to survive and function.

Case Study: Mercury Toxicity and Mitochondrial Damage

Patients with chronic mercury exposure often experience symptoms such as fatigue, muscle weakness, and cognitive impairment. Research has shown that mercury binds to proteins in the mitochondria, disrupting ATP production and leading to energy depletion in cells, particularly in the brain and muscles. This mechanism explains why mercury poisoning often manifests as neurological and muscular symptoms.

4. **Calcium Signalling and Neurotoxicity**

Heavy metals like lead and mercury interfere with calcium signalling, which is crucial for normal neuronal function. Calcium ions help transmit signals between neurons, and any disruption in this process can lead to impaired cognitive function, memory loss, and behavioural changes.

Analogy: Calcium signalling is like the "telecommunication system" of the brain, allowing neurons to communicate. Heavy metals act as "signal jammers," causing miscommunication and chaos in the brain.

Case Study: Lead-Induced Cognitive Decline in Children

Lead exposure in children has been associated with lower IQ scores, attention deficits, and behavioural problems. Lead disrupts calcium signalling in the developing brain, interfering with synapse formation and neurotransmitter release. This disruption results in long-term cognitive deficits, which may persist into adulthood.

These cellular and molecular mechanisms illustrate how heavy metals can cause a wide range of health issues, from anaemia and organ damage to cancer and neurological impairment. Even low levels of exposure, sustained over long periods, can lead to significant health consequences due to the cumulative nature of heavy metal toxicity.

Chronic vs. Acute Exposure

The health effects of heavy metals depend not only on the type of metal but also on the duration and intensity of exposure. Understanding the differences between chronic and acute exposure is essential for diagnosing and managing heavy metal toxicity.

1. **Acute Exposure**
   Acute exposure occurs when a person is exposed to a high dose of a heavy metal over a short period, usually leading to immediate and severe symptoms. This type of exposure is often the result of industrial accidents, ingestion of contaminated food or water, or use of certain products (e.g., mercury thermometers). Symptoms of acute exposure can include nausea, vomiting, abdominal pain, muscle spasms, and, in severe cases, organ failure and death.
   Analogy: Acute exposure is like a "sudden storm" that causes immediate damage. The body is overwhelmed by a high dose of the toxin, leading to rapid onset of symptoms.

   Case Study: Arsenic Poisoning from Contaminated Food

   A family in a rural community developed severe gastrointestinal symptoms, including vomiting and diarrhoea, after consuming rice from a local supplier. Investigations revealed that the rice was contaminated with high levels of arsenic, likely due to improper storage and the use of arsenic-based pesticides. Several family members were hospitalised, and one elderly member died from acute arsenic poisoning. This case highlights the dangers of acute exposure to heavy metals through food.

2. **Chronic Exposure**
   Chronic exposure occurs when a person is exposed to low levels of a heavy metal over an extended period, such as months or years. The cumulative nature of chronic exposure makes it particularly insidious. Heavy metals build up in tissues and organs, gradually causing damage that may not be immediately noticeable. Symptoms of chronic exposure can be vague and

include fatigue, memory loss, muscle pain, and general malaise. Because these symptoms overlap with many other conditions, chronic heavy metal toxicity is often misdiagnosed or overlooked.

Analogy: Chronic exposure is like "a slow drip" of poison— gradually accumulating in the body until it reaches a tipping point, where symptoms become apparent and irreversible damage is done.

Case Study: Chronic Lead Exposure in Urban Environments

A middle-aged man living in an older urban neighbourhood began experiencing unexplained fatigue, headaches, and irritability. Blood tests revealed elevated lead levels. It was later discovered that the soil around his home was contaminated with lead from years of industrial emissions and the use of leaded gasoline. Despite living in the area for decades, it took years for his symptoms to manifest clearly. This case illustrates how chronic exposure to low levels of heavy metals can lead to subtle but harmful health effects over time.

3. **Vulnerable Populations and Long-Term Consequences**
   Certain populations are more vulnerable to the effects of both acute and chronic heavy metal exposure. Children, pregnant women, and individuals with pre-existing health conditions are particularly at risk. For example, lead exposure in pregnant women can result in miscarriage, preterm birth, or developmental issues in the foetus.
4. **Analogy:** Vulnerable populations are like "dry sponges" that absorb toxins more readily. The health consequences for these groups can be more severe and long-lasting.

Case Study: Mercury Exposure in Pregnant Women
A pregnant woman who regularly consumed large amounts of fish was found to have elevated mercury levels in her blood. Her child, born prematurely, displayed symptoms of developmental delays and learning difficulties. Mercury's ability

to cross the placental barrier and its impact on fetal brain development makes it particularly dangerous for pregnant women.

Summary

Chapter 7 explores the complex mechanisms through which heavy metals cause damage at the cellular and molecular levels. From disrupting enzyme function to inducing oxidative stress, the toxic effects of heavy metals permeate every aspect of human biology. By distinguishing between acute and chronic exposure, the chapter highlights the diverse ways in which heavy metals can impact health, depending on the dose and duration of exposure.

Through detailed case studies and vivid analogies, this chapter provides a comprehensive understanding of why heavy metals are so harmful and how they contribute to a wide range of health issues. The next chapters will delve into the systemic health impacts of heavy metal exposure, further illustrating the far-reaching consequences of these toxic substances

Summary: Mechanisms of Toxicity

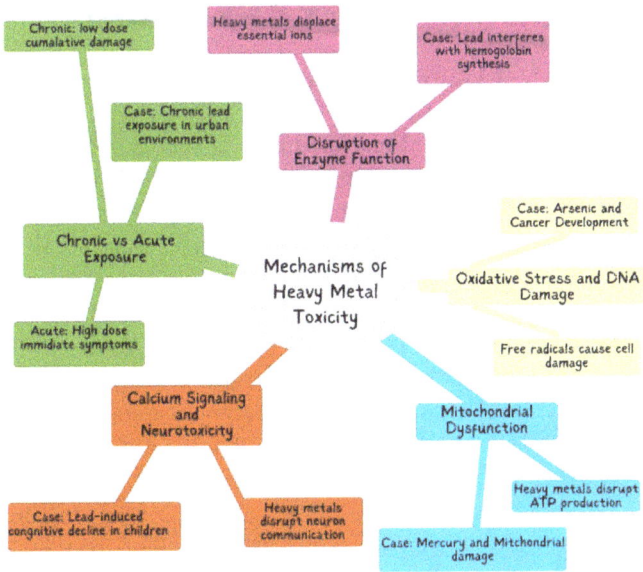

Chronic: low dose cumalative damage

Heavy metals displace essential ions

Case: Lead interferes with hemogolobin synthesis

Case: Chronic lead exposure in urban environments

Disruption of Enzyme Function

Chronic vs Acute Exposure

Mechanisms of Heavy Metal Toxicity

Case: Arsenic and Cancer Development

Oxidative Stress and DNA Damage

Acute: High dose immidiate symptoms

Free radicals cause cell damage

Calcium Signaling and Neurotoxicity

Mitochondrial Dysfunction

Heavy metals disrupt ATP production

Case: Lead-induced congnitive decline in children

Heavy metals disrupt neuron communication

Case: Mercury and Mitchondrial damage

Chapter 8: Systemic Health Impacts of Heavy Metals

Neurological Damage

The nervous system is highly susceptible to damage from heavy metal exposure, as many metals can cross the blood-brain barrier and accumulate in the brain. This accumulation can result in a range of neurological symptoms, from subtle cognitive impairments to severe neurodegenerative diseases.

1. **Lead and Neurodevelopmental Disorders**
   Lead is particularly harmful to the developing brain, making children one of the most vulnerable populations. Even low levels of lead exposure can interfere with the development of synapses and neurotransmitter release, leading to reduced cognitive function, behavioural problems, and learning disabilities. The damage caused by lead exposure is often irreversible, making early intervention and prevention crucial.
   Analogy: Lead exposure in children is like "a faulty wiring system" in a house — the brain's circuits don't connect properly, leading to miscommunication and power shortages.

   Case Study: The Flint Water Crisis

   In 2014, the city of Flint, Michigan, switched its water supply to the Flint River. The river water was highly corrosive and leached lead from old pipes into the water supply. Thousands of residents, including many children, were exposed to high levels of lead. The effects on children's health were profound, with an increase in developmental disorders, behavioural issues, and cognitive deficits. The Flint Water Crisis became a national symbol of the dangers of lead exposure and the devastating impact it can have on communities.

2. **Mercury and Neurotoxicity**

Mercury, particularly in its organic form (methylmercury), is a potent neurotoxin. It interferes with neurotransmitter function and disrupts cellular communication within the brain. Chronic mercury exposure can lead to symptoms such as tremors, memory loss, and mood disturbances. In severe cases, it can result in permanent damage to the central nervous system.

Analogy: Mercury acts like a "saboteur" in the brain's communication network, severing connections and distorting signals.

Case Study: Mercury Poisoning in Minamata Bay

The Minamata disease outbreak in Japan, caused by industrial mercury contamination, resulted in severe neurological symptoms in affected individuals, including loss of motor control, cognitive impairment, and speech difficulties. Many children born to affected mothers exhibited developmental delays and severe congenital disabilities. This case highlights the devastating effects of mercury on the nervous system, particularly in vulnerable populations such as pregnant women and children.

3. **Arsenic and Cognitive Impairment**

Chronic exposure to arsenic, often through contaminated drinking water, has been linked to cognitive decline and an increased risk of neurodegenerative diseases such as Alzheimer's and Parkinson's. Arsenic induces oxidative stress and inflammation in the brain, which can lead to neuron death and the formation of protein aggregates associated with neurodegeneration.

Analogy: Arsenic exposure is like a "rusting process" in the brain, slowly corroding neurons and weakening the structural integrity of the nervous system.

Case Study: Arsenic in Drinking Water in Bangladesh

In Bangladesh, millions of people have been exposed to high levels of arsenic in their drinking water. Studies have shown that affected individuals have a higher incidence of cognitive decline and memory loss. This widespread public health issue has drawn international attention and led to efforts to provide safer drinking water solutions to impacted communities.

Cardiovascular and Renal Issues

Heavy metals can also have profound effects on the cardiovascular and renal systems, leading to hypertension, heart disease, kidney damage, and even failure. The kidneys and heart are particularly vulnerable because they filter and pump blood, making them susceptible to heavy metal accumulation.

1. **Cardiovascular Effects**
   Lead and cadmium are known to increase the risk of hypertension and cardiovascular disease. These metals cause oxidative stress and endothelial dysfunction, which impair blood vessel function and promote the build-up of plaque in arteries (atherosclerosis). Long-term exposure can lead to an increased risk of heart attacks, strokes, and other cardiovascular events.
   Analogy: Heavy metals in the cardiovascular system are like "sand in a machine" — they grind down the smooth functioning of the heart and blood vessels, causing blockages and breakdowns.

   Case Study: Lead Exposure and Hypertension in Urban Populations

   Studies have shown that people living in urban areas with high levels of lead in the environment are more likely to develop hypertension. One study conducted in New York City found a strong correlation between elevated blood lead levels and high blood pressure, particularly in middle-aged and elderly residents.

The increased cardiovascular risk in these populations has been linked to long-term exposure to lead from air pollution, old plumbing systems, and industrial emissions.

2. **Renal Effects**
   The kidneys are the body's primary detoxification organs, filtering out waste and toxins from the blood. Heavy metals such as cadmium, lead, and mercury accumulate in the kidneys, leading to nephrotoxicity. Chronic exposure can cause a decline in kidney function, proteinuria (excess protein in the urine), and even kidney failure.
   Analogy: Heavy metals act like "clogged filters" in the kidneys, disrupting their ability to cleanse the body and leading to a toxic build-up of waste.

   Case Study: Cadmium Exposure and Kidney Disease in Battery Factory Workers

   Battery factory workers exposed to cadmium dust are at high risk for developing kidney disease. Prolonged exposure to cadmium has been shown to cause tubular damage, leading to proteinuria and chronic kidney disease. Studies on these workers have demonstrated a direct link between occupational cadmium exposure and progressive kidney dysfunction.

Impacts on Reproductive Health

Heavy metals can have serious implications for reproductive health, affecting fertility, pregnancy outcomes, and developmental health in offspring. Metals such as lead, mercury, and arsenic are known to disrupt hormonal balance, impair sperm and egg quality, and cause birth defects.

1. **Effects on Fertility**
   Lead and mercury can interfere with the endocrine system, leading to hormonal imbalances that impair reproductive function in both men and women. In men, these metals can

reduce sperm count and motility, while in women, they can disrupt the menstrual cycle and reduce ovarian function.

Analogy: Heavy metals in the reproductive system are like "roadblocks" that prevent the natural flow of hormonal signals and reproductive processes.

Case Study: Lead Exposure and Infertility in Men

Studies have shown that male workers exposed to lead in industries such as painting and battery manufacturing have lower sperm counts and reduced fertility. One study of lead-exposed factory workers found that nearly 40% of the men had abnormal sperm parameters, which were linked to high blood lead levels. This case highlights the detrimental impact of lead on male reproductive health.

2. **Effects on Pregnancy and Fetal Development**

   Heavy metals can cross the placental barrier, exposing the developing fetus to toxins that can cause birth defects, low birth weight, and developmental delays. Mercury is particularly harmful as it can accumulate in the fetal brain, disrupting neurodevelopment.

   Analogy: Heavy metals act like "silent intruders" during pregnancy, crossing the protective barrier of the placenta and interfering with the delicate process of fetal development.

Case Study: Methylmercury and Birth Defects in the Minamata Outbreak

In the Minamata disease outbreak in Japan, pregnant women who consumed mercury-contaminated fish gave birth to children with severe neurological disorders and congenital defects. Many of these children exhibited cerebral palsy-like symptoms, including impaired motor function and intellectual disabilities. This case underscores the profound impact of heavy metals on fetal development and the need for stringent protections for pregnant women.

Summary

Chapter 8 explores the systemic health impacts of heavy metal exposure, focusing on the neurological, cardiovascular, renal, and reproductive systems. The chapter highlights how metals such as lead, mercury, cadmium, and arsenic disrupt normal physiological processes, leading to a range of health issues, from cognitive impairment and hypertension to infertility and birth defects.

Detailed case studies, including the Flint Water Crisis and the Minamata disease outbreak, provide real-world examples of how these toxic substances affect vulnerable populations. Through vivid analogies and case histories, this chapter emphasises the far-reaching consequences of heavy metal exposure, setting the stage for understanding the challenges of diagnosis and treatment, which will be discussed in the following chapters.

Summary: Systemic Health Impacts of Heavy Metals

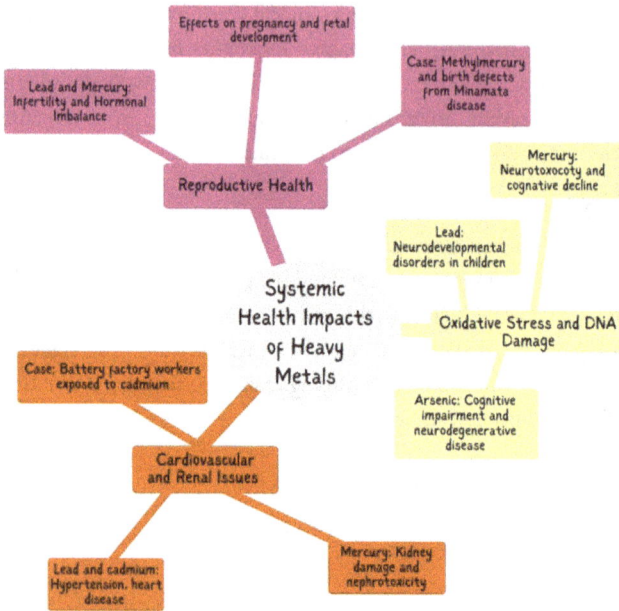

Effects on pregnancy and fetal development

Case: Methylmercury and birth defects from Minamata disease

Lead and Mercury: Infertility and Hormonal Imbalance

Reproductive Health

Mercury: Neurotoxocity and cognative decline

Lead: Neurodevelopmental disorders in children

Systemic Health Impacts of Heavy Metals

Oxidative Stress and DNA Damage

Case: Battery factory workers exposed to cadmium

Arsenic: Cognitive impairment and neurodegenerative disease

Cardiovascular and Renal Issues

Lead and cadmium: Hypertension, heart disease

Mercury: Kidney damage and nephrotoxicity

Chapter 9: The Silent Epidemic – Why Heavy Metal Toxicity Is Often Missed

Why Heavy Metal Toxicity Is Often Missed

Heavy metal toxicity is often referred to as a "silent epidemic" because it frequently goes undiagnosed or misdiagnosed. The insidious nature of heavy metal exposure, combined with vague and non-specific symptoms, makes it difficult for healthcare professionals to identify. This leads to prolonged suffering and can exacerbate chronic health conditions if not properly addressed.

1. **Subtle and Non-Specific Symptoms**
   Heavy metal toxicity manifests in a wide array of symptoms, many of which mimic other conditions. Fatigue, headaches, joint pain, digestive issues, and cognitive disturbances are common complaints. Because these symptoms overlap with conditions such as chronic fatigue syndrome, fibromyalgia, autoimmune disorders, and psychiatric illnesses, heavy metal toxicity is often overlooked.
   Analogy: Heavy metal toxicity is like a "chameleon" — it takes on the appearance of other diseases, blending in and eluding detection.

Case Study: Misdiagnosis of Chronic Mercury Poisoning as Depression

A 42-year-old woman began experiencing severe fatigue, memory loss, and irritability. She was initially diagnosed with depression and prescribed antidepressants. When her symptoms failed to improve, further tests revealed elevated mercury levels, likely from her amalgam dental fillings. Her condition improved dramatically after undergoing a mercury detoxification protocol. This case underscores how easily heavy metal toxicity can be mistaken for psychiatric conditions.

2. **Lack of Routine Screening and Testing**
Conventional medical practice does not typically include heavy metal testing as part of standard diagnostic procedures. Most doctors are not trained to consider heavy metal exposure as a potential cause of chronic symptoms, and specialised tests like hair analysis, urine challenge tests, or blood plasma analysis are not commonly ordered. As a result, patients can go for years without discovering the true cause of their health issues.
Analogy: Detecting heavy metal toxicity is like "finding a needle in a haystack" — without the right tools and knowledge, it is nearly impossible to identify the root cause.

Case Study: Missed Lead Poisoning in Children

A family living in an old house noticed that their three-year-old son was experiencing developmental delays and frequent irritability. Their paediatrician attributed the symptoms to behavioural issues. It wasn't until a routine check-up included a blood test that the child's elevated lead levels were discovered. The cause? Peeling lead-based paint in their 100-year-old home. This case highlights how routine screening could have caught the problem earlier, preventing months of unnecessary suffering.

3. **Subclinical and Cumulative Nature of Heavy Metal Toxicity**
Heavy metal toxicity often develops slowly over time. Low-level exposure accumulates in the body's tissues, and symptoms may not become apparent until a tipping point is reached. This subclinical presentation makes it difficult to establish a direct link between exposure and symptoms. Additionally, because the body can store heavy metals in bones, organs, and fat tissues, standard blood tests may not reveal the full extent of toxicity.
Analogy: Heavy metal toxicity is like a "time bomb" ticking away quietly in the body. The effects may not be felt

immediately, but they build up over time, leading to a sudden and severe manifestation of symptoms once the body can no longer compensate.

Case Study: Chronic Arsenic Exposure in Well Water

Residents of a small rural town consumed water from a well contaminated with low levels of arsenic for decades. Over the years, many residents developed symptoms like numbness, skin lesions, and chronic fatigue. It wasn't until several cases of skin cancer emerged that health authorities tested the water and discovered arsenic contamination. By then, the cumulative exposure had already taken a significant toll on the community's health.

Challenges in Diagnosis

The diagnosis of heavy metal toxicity presents unique challenges for both patients and healthcare providers. Because the symptoms can be attributed to a wide range of other conditions, and because standard testing methods have limitations, many cases remain undiagnosed or misdiagnosed.

1. **Limitations of Standard Blood Tests**
   Standard blood tests can detect only recent or acute exposure to heavy metals. Since many metals accumulate in tissues such as the liver, kidneys, bones, and brain, blood levels may not reflect the body's total heavy metal burden. For example, lead can be stored in bones for years, and a blood test may show normal lead levels even in cases of significant long-term exposure. Similarly, mercury can accumulate in the brain and may not appear in routine blood tests.
   Analogy: Testing for heavy metals in the blood is like "checking the surface of a lake" for pollution — it gives a snapshot of the current state but doesn't reveal the contaminants settled at the bottom.

Case Study: Normal Blood Levels, Hidden Toxicity

A middle-aged man with chronic fatigue and muscle weakness underwent a standard blood test for heavy metals, which came back normal. However, after years of unexplained symptoms, he pursued a more comprehensive test — a urine challenge test — which revealed high levels of mercury and cadmium. This case illustrates how standard testing can fail to capture the full extent of heavy metal toxicity.

2. **Reliability and Accessibility of Diagnostic Tests**

Advanced diagnostic methods, such as hair mineral analysis, urine provocation tests, and the Oligoscan, can provide a better picture of heavy metal toxicity. However, these tests are not widely available, and there is controversy over their accuracy and interpretation. Hair analysis, for instance, can show past exposure but may be affected by external contamination. Urine provocation tests require the use of chelating agents, which can cause side effects and are not suitable for everyone. As a result, many doctors are hesitant to use these tests, and patients are left with few options for definitive diagnosis.

Analogy: Diagnosing heavy metal toxicity is like "trying to see through fog" — even with advanced tools, it's challenging to get a clear picture.

Case Study: The Controversy of Hair Analysis in Diagnosing Heavy Metal Toxicity

A woman experiencing unexplained hair loss and skin rashes decided to get a hair mineral analysis, which revealed elevated levels of arsenic. However, her doctor dismissed the results, attributing them to potential contamination from hair dyes. It wasn't until a urine test confirmed the elevated levels that her diagnosis was accepted, and treatment began. This case highlights the scepticism surrounding alternative diagnostic methods and the difficulty in obtaining a definitive diagnosis.

3. Misdiagnosis and Inadequate Treatment

Because heavy metal toxicity is not commonly considered in conventional medical practice, patients are often misdiagnosed with other conditions. This can lead to ineffective treatments that fail to address the underlying cause. Misdiagnosis is particularly common in cases of neurological or psychiatric symptoms, where heavy metals can mimic conditions such as anxiety, depression, and even early-onset dementia.

Analogy: Misdiagnosis is like "chasing shadows" — treating the symptoms without understanding the root cause.

Case Study: Mercury Toxicity Misdiagnosed as Early-Onset Dementia

A 50-year-old woman began experiencing memory loss, confusion, and tremors. She was diagnosed with early-onset dementia and prescribed medication, but her condition continued to deteriorate. Frustrated with the lack of improvement, her family sought a second opinion. A comprehensive evaluation, including urine and hair analysis, revealed high levels of mercury, likely from seafood consumption and dental amalgams. After undergoing a chelation therapy protocol, her cognitive symptoms improved significantly, confirming that her "dementia" had been caused by mercury toxicity.

Summary

Chapter 9 delves into why heavy metal toxicity is often missed, misdiagnosed, or misunderstood. With vague symptoms, limitations in standard testing, and the cumulative nature of toxicity, heavy metal poisoning is a "silent epidemic" that eludes detection. The chapter explores the challenges in diagnosing heavy metal toxicity and provides real-world case studies to illustrate the difficulties patients face in getting an accurate diagnosis.

By highlighting the complexities and misconceptions surrounding heavy metal diagnosis, this chapter emphasises the need for increased awareness, better diagnostic tools, and a more holistic approach to healthcare. This sets the stage for understanding how effective detection and treatment strategies can be implemented, which will be discussed in subsequent chapters.

Summary: The Silent Epidemic – Why Heavy Metal Toxicity Is Often Missed

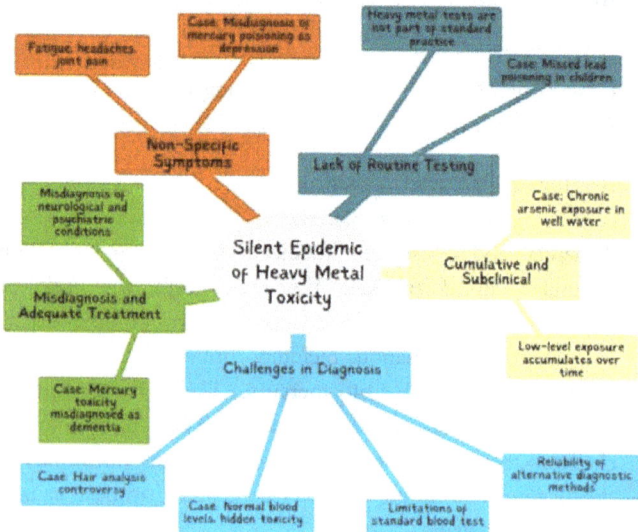

Chapter 10: Traditional Diagnostic Methods

Blood and Plasma Testing

Blood and plasma tests are often the first step in evaluating heavy metal exposure, especially in acute cases. These tests measure the concentration of heavy metals, such as lead, mercury, arsenic, and cadmium, in the bloodstream. However, while blood tests are useful for detecting recent or high-level exposure, they have significant limitations when it comes to assessing chronic or long-term exposure.

1. **Strengths of Blood and Plasma Testing**
   Blood tests are effective at identifying acute or recent heavy metal exposure, particularly in cases where symptoms have emerged rapidly following a known exposure event. For example, if a child ingests lead paint chips or an industrial worker is exposed to mercury vapours, a blood test can confirm elevated levels of these metals. Blood tests are widely accessible and relatively inexpensive, making them a common choice in emergency situations.
   Analogy: Blood tests are like "sniffer dogs" that detect toxic metals immediately after exposure but can't follow the trail once the metals have left the bloodstream.

   Case Study: Lead Poisoning Detected in a Child

   A three-year-old child in an old home began experiencing abdominal pain, irritability, and developmental delays. A blood test revealed elevated lead levels, prompting the removal of lead-based paint from the home and initiation of chelation therapy. The blood test successfully identified the source of acute exposure, leading to timely intervention.

2. **Limitations of Blood and Plasma Testing**

Heavy metals such as lead, mercury, and cadmium tend to accumulate in tissues rather than remain in the blood. After initial exposure, these metals are sequestered in bones, organs, and fat tissues, making them difficult to detect with standard blood tests. For example, lead can be stored in bones for decades and only released back into the bloodstream under certain conditions, such as pregnancy or bone fractures. Thus, a patient may have significant heavy metal toxicity but present with normal blood levels.

Analogy: Blood tests are like "checking the surface of an iceberg"—only a small fraction of the total heavy metal burden is visible, while the majority remains hidden beneath the surface.

Case Study: Normal Blood Lead Levels Despite Chronic Exposure

A 45-year-old man experiencing unexplained fatigue and joint pain had a standard blood test for heavy metals, which came back normal. However, a bone biopsy later revealed high levels of lead accumulation, likely due to long-term exposure from old plumbing in his home. This case illustrates how blood tests can fail to detect chronic heavy metal toxicity, leading to missed diagnoses and prolonged suffering.

3. **Challenges with Mercury and Arsenic Detection**

Mercury and arsenic can also pose challenges for blood testing. Inorganic mercury may be present in blood for only a short time before being deposited in organs like the kidneys and brain. Similarly, arsenic levels can fluctuate rapidly and may not reflect chronic exposure through drinking water or food. Therefore, while blood tests are helpful in acute scenarios, they are not reliable for long-term exposure evaluation.

Analogy: Blood tests for mercury and arsenic are like trying to catch a "fleeting shadow" — the metals pass through quickly and can be missed entirely.

Urine and Hair Analysis

Urine and hair analysis offer alternative ways to assess heavy metal exposure, particularly for chronic or long-term toxicity. These methods provide insights into the body's overall heavy metal burden and can reveal exposure that blood tests might miss. However, they also come with their own set of limitations and controversies.

1. **Urine Testing**
   Urine tests measure the concentration of heavy metals excreted by the body. They are especially useful for detecting chronic exposure and can be enhanced with a urine challenge test. In this test, a chelating agent such as EDTA or DMSA is administered to "pull" metals from tissues into the bloodstream, where they are excreted in urine. This method provides a better picture of the total body burden of metals like lead, mercury, and cadmium. **Analogy:** Urine tests are like "flushing out the pipes" to see what has been building up over time — the more that is flushed out, the more is revealed about what's hidden inside.

   Case Study: Urine Challenge Test Reveals Hidden Lead Toxicity

   A 55-year-old woman suffering from chronic headaches and muscle pain underwent a standard blood test for heavy metals, which showed no abnormalities. However, after her doctor administered a urine challenge test, her urine showed high levels of lead, confirming chronic lead toxicity. The urine test provided a clearer picture of her long-term exposure and led to the initiation of chelation therapy.

2. **Strengths and Weaknesses of Urine Testing**
   Urine testing can reveal metals that are actively being excreted, but it doesn't always reflect metals stored in tissues. Furthermore, the use of chelating agents in challenge tests can mobilise metals too quickly, leading to temporary spikes in toxicity and adverse effects. Because of this, urine challenge

tests should be conducted cautiously, under medical supervision.

Analogy: Urine tests are like "cleaning out a clogged drain" — they show what's being released but don't reveal the full extent of what's stuck in the system.

3. **Hair Analysis**

Hair analysis measures the concentration of heavy metals in hair strands, which can reflect long-term exposure. Because hair grows slowly, it can provide a historical record of exposure over months or even years. Hair analysis is particularly useful for detecting metals like mercury and arsenic, which are readily incorporated into hair strands. However, hair analysis is subject to contamination from external sources, such as hair products or environmental pollutants, which can lead to misleading results. **Analogy:** Hair analysis is like "reading a tree's growth rings" — it shows past exposure over time but can be distorted by external factors.

Case Study: Hair Analysis Uncovers Mercury Toxicity in a Dental Worker

A dental hygienist experiencing tremors and mood swings underwent hair analysis, which showed high levels of mercury. The source was traced to her occupational exposure to mercury-containing amalgam fillings. The hair analysis provided a clear link between her symptoms and her work environment, prompting workplace safety changes and treatment.

4. **Controversies and Challenges in Hair Analysis**

Hair analysis is not universally accepted due to concerns about reliability and interpretation. Variations in hair washing, exposure to dyes, and even the location of hair sampling can affect results. Critics argue that without strict standardisation, hair analysis can produce false positives or negatives, complicating the diagnostic process.

Analogy: Hair analysis can be like "trying to read a story written in sand" — the results can be influenced by many external factors, making it difficult to draw definitive conclusions.

5. **Combining Diagnostic Methods**

   Because no single test provides a complete picture of heavy metal toxicity, a combination of diagnostic methods is often necessary. Blood, urine, and hair tests each provide different insights, and together, they can help build a more comprehensive understanding of a patient's heavy metal exposure. This integrative approach is particularly valuable when trying to determine the source, extent, and duration of exposure.

   Analogy: Combining diagnostic tests is like "assembling pieces of a puzzle" — each test contributes a piece, and only when combined do they reveal the full picture.

Summary

Chapter 10 explores traditional diagnostic methods for detecting heavy metal toxicity, including blood and plasma tests, urine tests, and hair analysis. While blood tests are useful for identifying recent or acute exposure, they fall short in detecting chronic or long-term toxicity. Urine tests, especially when combined with chelating agents, can provide insights into the body's overall metal burden, while hair analysis offers a historical record of exposure.

The chapter highlights the strengths and limitations of each method through detailed case studies and analogies, emphasising the need for a multifaceted approach to diagnosis. Understanding these diagnostic methods lays the groundwork for exploring more advanced and emerging techniques, which will be covered in the following chapter.

Summary: Traditional Diagnostic Methods

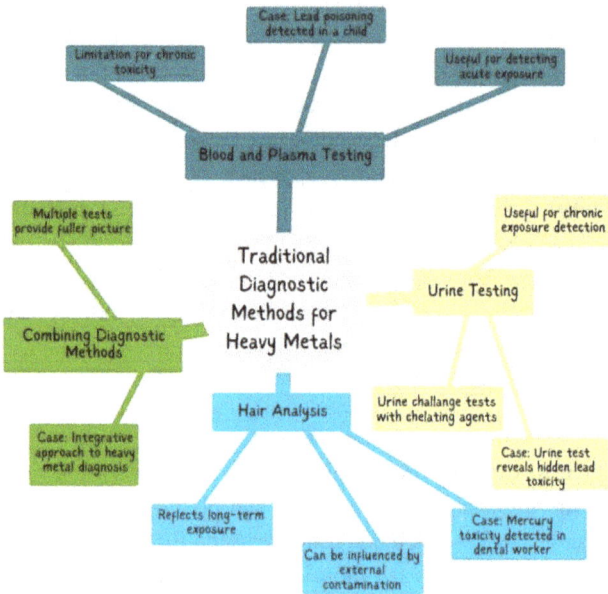

Chapter 11: Advanced Diagnostic Techniques

Oligoscan: Pros and Cons

The Oligoscan is a relatively new diagnostic tool used to evaluate heavy metal toxicity and mineral imbalances. It utilises spectrophotometry technology, a non-invasive method that measures the absorbance of light wavelengths by elements in the body. By scanning the tissues, typically on the palm of the hand, the Oligoscan can provide immediate data on heavy metal levels and essential mineral concentrations. While it offers several advantages, it also has limitations that make its use somewhat controversial.

1. **How the Oligoscan Works**
   The Oligoscan emits light wavelengths that interact with the elements present in the skin. Each element absorbs a specific wavelength of light, allowing the device to measure the concentration of various heavy metals and minerals. This information is then processed through an algorithm to produce a report that shows the levels of toxic metals like lead, mercury, arsenic, and cadmium, as well as essential minerals such as calcium, magnesium, and zinc.
   Analogy: The Oligoscan is like a "metal detector" for the body, scanning for both beneficial and harmful metals in a matter of minutes.

   Case Study: Immediate Assessment with Oligoscan

   A 40-year-old woman experiencing chronic fatigue and muscle weakness used the Oligoscan to check for heavy metal toxicity. The scan revealed high levels of mercury and low levels of essential minerals like magnesium and calcium. This information prompted her to undergo further testing and initiate a detoxification protocol. The Oligoscan's rapid results allowed her to start treatment much sooner than with conventional tests, which could have taken weeks to complete.

2. **Strengths of the Oligoscan**
   a. **Non-Invasive and Painless:** The Oligoscan doesn't require blood draws or urine collection, making it an attractive option for patients who are averse to needles or have difficulty providing samples.
   b. **Immediate Results:** Unlike traditional tests that may take days or weeks, the Oligoscan provides results within minutes, allowing for real-time discussion and treatment planning.
   c. **Broad Screening Capability:** The device can measure both heavy metals and essential minerals, providing a more comprehensive view of the body's metal and mineral status.

3. **Limitations and Controversies**
   a. **Lack of Standardisation:** The Oligoscan's results can be affected by skin hydration, pigmentation, and thickness, leading to variability in measurements. This lack of standardisation makes it difficult to compare results between different individuals or sessions.
   b. **Limited Validation and Scientific Backing:** Critics argue that the Oligoscan lacks robust clinical validation. There is limited peer-reviewed research supporting its accuracy and reliability, leading to scepticism among healthcare professionals.
   c. **Dependence on Algorithms:** The Oligoscan's reliance on proprietary algorithms raises concerns about the objectivity of the results, as these algorithms are not publicly accessible or independently verified.

Analogy: The Oligoscan is like "a high-tech guesser" — while it can provide useful insights, its results should be interpreted with caution and confirmed with more established diagnostic methods.

Case Study: False Positive for Cadmium Exposure

A 35-year-old man used the Oligoscan, which indicated dangerously high levels of cadmium. Concerned, he underwent further testing through blood and urine analysis, both of which showed normal cadmium levels. It was later discovered that his recent use of a cadmium-containing ointment had interfered with the scan's accuracy. This case demonstrates the potential for false positives and the importance of corroborating Oligoscan results with other diagnostic methods.

Emerging Technologies in Metal Detection

As understanding of heavy metal toxicity has grown, so too has the development of more sophisticated diagnostic techniques. Emerging technologies aim to provide more accurate, reliable, and comprehensive assessments of heavy metal exposure and its health impacts. Some of these advanced methods include tissue biopsies, intracellular mineral analysis, and cutting-edge imaging technologies.

1. **Tissue Biopsies and Mineral Analysis**
   Tissue biopsies involve sampling small amounts of tissues like skin, hair, or nails to measure heavy metal concentrations. These samples can reflect long-term exposure better than blood or urine tests. For example, bone biopsies are considered the gold standard for assessing chronic lead exposure, as lead can accumulate in bones for decades. Similarly, hair analysis can provide a timeline of heavy metal exposure over several months. **Analogy:** Tissue biopsies are like "core samples" taken from the Earth — they provide a historical record of exposure and can reveal the extent of contamination over time.

Case Study: Bone Biopsy for Chronic Lead Toxicity

A middle-aged man with a history of occupational exposure to lead underwent a bone biopsy after experiencing persistent joint pain and anaemia. The biopsy revealed lead levels ten times higher than normal, confirming chronic toxicity. This led to a treatment plan that included chelation therapy and dietary modifications.

2. **Intracellular Mineral Analysis**

Intracellular mineral analysis measures the concentration of metals inside cells, rather than in extracellular fluids like blood or urine. This technique provides a more accurate picture of how metals are affecting cellular function, particularly in organs like the liver, kidneys, and brain. Intracellular analysis can be conducted using advanced microscopy techniques or through the use of biomarkers that indicate cellular metal concentration. **Analogy:** Intracellular analysis is like "peering inside a cell's machinery" to see how it is affected by toxic metals, providing a more detailed view of cellular health.

Case Study: Intracellular Mercury Analysis in a Patient with Cognitive Decline

A 60-year-old woman with unexplained cognitive decline underwent intracellular mercury analysis, which revealed high concentrations of mercury in her brain cells. This result explained her symptoms and led to the diagnosis of mercury toxicity. Following treatment, her cognitive function improved, demonstrating the value of this advanced diagnostic approach.

3. **Cutting-Edge Imaging Technologies**

Advanced imaging technologies, such as magnetic resonance imaging (MRI) and positron emission tomography (PET), are being explored for their ability to detect heavy metal deposits in the brain and other organs. For example, MRI can visualise the accumulation of iron and other metals in the brain, which is particularly useful for studying neurodegenerative diseases like Alzheimer's and Parkinson's. PET scans, on the other hand, can be used to study the effects of heavy metals on brain function and metabolism. **Analogy:** Advanced imaging is like "shining a spotlight" on hidden metal deposits in the body, allowing doctors to see where and how metals are affecting health.

Case Study: MRI Detects Iron Accumulation in a Parkinson's Patient

A 70-year-old man with Parkinson's disease underwent an MRI scan, which revealed excessive iron deposits in specific regions of his brain. This finding supported the theory that iron accumulation contributes to the neurodegenerative process in Parkinson's. The MRI results prompted further research and personalised treatment strategies aimed at reducing iron levels and slowing disease progression.

4. **Biomonitoring and Nanotechnology-Based Tests**
Biomonitoring involves measuring the levels of metals and other toxins in biological samples like blood, urine, and tissues over time to track exposure trends. Advances in nanotechnology have led to the development of sensors that can detect heavy metals at extremely low concentrations, providing highly sensitive and specific results. These sensors can be incorporated into wearable devices, allowing continuous monitoring of metal exposure in real time.
Analogy: Biomonitoring and nanotechnology are like "personal environmental watchdogs," constantly alerting to the presence of toxic metals before they reach harmful levels.

Case Study: Real-Time Lead Detection with a Wearable Sensor

Researchers developed a wearable sensor that could detect lead in sweat. When worn by children in high-risk areas, the sensor successfully identified low-level lead exposure, prompting early intervention and preventing more severe health outcomes. This technology represents a significant leap forward in the prevention and early detection of heavy metal toxicity.

Summary

Chapter 11 explores advanced diagnostic techniques for detecting heavy metal toxicity, including the Oligoscan, tissue biopsies, intracellular mineral analysis, and emerging imaging technologies. While these methods provide valuable insights into the body's heavy metal burden, each comes with its own set of strengths and limitations. Case studies and analogies illustrate how these tools can be used to diagnose both chronic and acute heavy metal exposure more accurately.

As the field of toxicology continues to evolve, these emerging technologies offer hope for more precise and personalised approaches to diagnosing and managing heavy metal toxicity. This chapter sets the stage for discussing how these diagnostic methods can inform effective treatment strategies, which will be covered in the following chapters.

Summary: Advanced Diagnostic Techniques

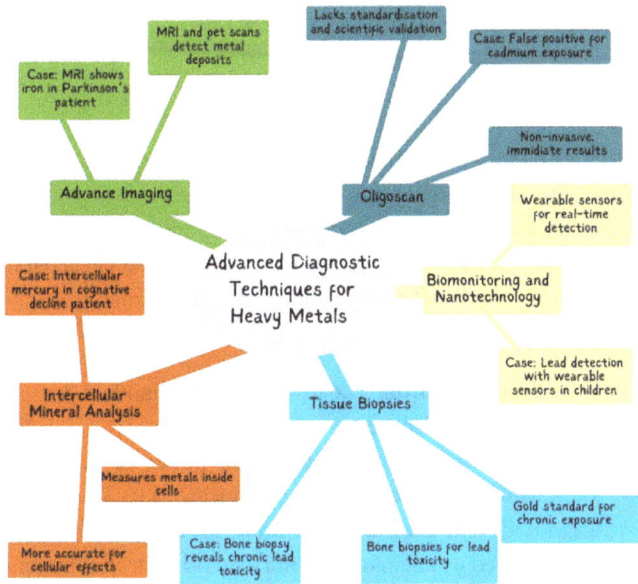

Advanced Diagnostic Techniques for Heavy Metals

Advance Imaging
- MRI and pet scans detect metal deposits
- Case: MRI shows iron in Parkinson's patient

Oligoscan
- Lacks standardisation and scientific validation
- Case: False positive for cadmium exposure
- Non-invasive, immidiate results

Biomonitoring and Nanotechnology
- Wearable sensors for real-time detection
- Case: Lead detection with wearable sensors in children

Intercellular Mineral Analysis
- Case: Intercellular mercury in cognative decline patient
- Measures metals inside cells
- More accurate for cellular effects

Tissue Biopsies
- Case: Bone biopsy reveals chronic lead toxicity
- Bone biopsies for lead toxicity
- Gold standard for chronic exposure

Chapter 12: Case Studies in Diagnosis

Misdiagnosed Cases and Lessons Learned

Heavy metal toxicity is often overlooked or misdiagnosed due to its complex presentation and non-specific symptoms. Misdiagnosis can lead to ineffective treatment and prolonged suffering. In this chapter, we'll explore several case studies that illustrate the challenges of diagnosing heavy metal toxicity and the lessons learned from these experiences.

1. **Case Study 1: Chronic Lead Poisoning Mistaken for Autoimmune Disease**

   Patient Profile: A 45-year-old woman presented with fatigue, joint pain, and cognitive impairment. She was initially diagnosed with rheumatoid arthritis, an autoimmune disease characterised by inflammation and joint pain. Despite treatment with anti-inflammatory medications, her symptoms continued to worsen.

   Misdiagnosis and Outcome: After two years of ineffective treatment, the patient sought a second opinion from a functional medicine practitioner, who recommended comprehensive heavy metal testing. The results revealed high levels of lead in her bones, likely due to childhood exposure from living in a home with lead-based paint. The patient's lead levels were undetectable in standard blood tests because the metal had been sequestered in her bones for decades. Once the correct diagnosis of chronic lead toxicity was made, she underwent chelation therapy and began to show significant improvement.

   Lesson Learned: Heavy metal toxicity should be considered in cases of unexplained joint pain and cognitive decline, especially when patients have a history of living in older homes or working in environments with potential lead exposure.

Chronic toxicity may not always be detected with standard blood tests, making comprehensive testing crucial.

2. **Case Study 2: Mercury Toxicity Misdiagnosed as Bipolar Disorder**

   Patient Profile: A 38-year-old man experienced sudden mood swings, anxiety, and severe irritability. He was diagnosed with bipolar disorder and prescribed mood stabilisers and antipsychotic medications. His condition did not improve, and he experienced worsening symptoms, including tremors and memory loss.

   Misdiagnosis and Outcome: Frustrated with the lack of progress, the patient sought help from an integrative psychiatrist, who suspected heavy metal toxicity. A hair mineral analysis and urine challenge test revealed high levels of mercury, likely due to his occupation as a dentist working with mercury-based amalgam fillings. Once the mercury was removed from his body through chelation and the amalgams were replaced with safer materials, his psychiatric symptoms resolved, and his cognitive function returned to normal.

   Lesson Learned: Heavy metal toxicity can mimic psychiatric disorders. When conventional treatments for mood disorders are ineffective, it is essential to rule out underlying toxicities, especially in patients with occupational exposure to mercury or other heavy metals.

3. **Case Study 3: Dr Chris Kresser's Personal Struggle with Mercury Toxicity**

   Patient Profile: Dr Chris Kresser, a respected functional medicine practitioner and health educator, began experiencing unexplained symptoms such as brain fog, fatigue, and digestive issues early in his career. Despite consulting numerous specialists, his symptoms were attributed to stress and dietary factors, and he was misdiagnosed with conditions ranging from irritable bowel syndrome (IBS) to chronic fatigue syndrome (CFS).

Misdiagnosis and Outcome: It wasn't until Dr Kresser sought help from a fellow functional medicine practitioner that comprehensive heavy metal testing was conducted. The tests revealed alarmingly high levels of mercury in his system. As a result of this finding, Dr Kresser was able to identify the source of his mercury exposure — regular consumption of large predatory fish like tuna and swordfish, which are known to accumulate high levels of methylmercury. He underwent a comprehensive mercury detoxification protocol, including dietary changes, chelation therapy, and supportive supplements. Within a few months, his symptoms began to improve, and he made a full recovery.

Lesson Learned: Dr Kresser's case highlights the importance of considering heavy metal toxicity in patients with vague, unexplained symptoms, particularly when they have a history of dietary habits or environmental exposure that could increase their risk. His experience underscores the need for greater awareness and training among healthcare professionals to recognise and diagnose heavy metal toxicity accurately.

4. **Case Study 4: Arsenic Poisoning Confused with Gastrointestinal Disorders**

   Patient Profile: A 60-year-old man with a history of gastrointestinal discomfort, weight loss, and skin lesions was diagnosed with irritable bowel syndrome (IBS). Over the next five years, his symptoms progressively worsened, and he developed peripheral neuropathy (numbness and tingling in his extremities).

   Misdiagnosis and Outcome: After multiple misdiagnoses, a specialist considered environmental toxin exposure as a potential cause and ordered a urine test for heavy metals. The test revealed high levels of arsenic, likely from contaminated well water in his rural hometown. With detoxification treatments and a switch to clean water, his gastrointestinal symptoms and neuropathy improved significantly.

Lesson Learned: Persistent gastrointestinal symptoms that do not respond to standard treatments should prompt testing for heavy metals, particularly in regions known for water contamination or in patients with unexplained skin changes or neurological symptoms.

Diagnostic Challenges Across Eras

The challenges of diagnosing heavy metal toxicity have changed over time as medical knowledge and diagnostic tools have advanced. In the past, heavy metal poisoning was often identified only after severe and obvious symptoms emerged. Today, the increased availability of diagnostic tests allows for earlier detection, but many hurdles remain.

1. **19th Century: Limited Diagnostic Awareness and Tools**
    During the 19th century, heavy metal toxicity was rarely recognised until it caused extreme symptoms, such as "Mad Hatter's disease" in hatmakers exposed to mercury or lead colic in industrial workers. The lack of understanding about the mechanisms of toxicity, combined with limited diagnostic tools, meant that heavy metal poisoning was often identified too late to prevent irreversible damage. Diagnoses were usually made based on obvious clinical presentations, such as severe tremors, abdominal pain, or neurological impairment.

    Case Example: In 19th-century England, a group of hatmakers suffering from tremors, confusion, and emotional instability were thought to be suffering from "occupational madness." It wasn't until years later that the connection between mercury exposure and neurological symptoms was established, leading to improved workplace safety standards.

2. **Early 20th Century: Advances in Testing but Limited Public Awareness**
    The early 20th century saw the development of basic laboratory tests for detecting metals like lead and mercury in blood and urine. However, these tests were not widely available, and

awareness of heavy metal toxicity among healthcare professionals and the public remained low. Many cases of poisoning were attributed to other conditions, and only severe cases with clear occupational links were properly diagnosed.

Case Example: In the 1920s, a group of American factory workers exposed to cadmium in battery production experienced kidney damage and bone pain. The connection to cadmium toxicity was not made until a decade later, as the use of cadmium had only recently been introduced in manufacturing. This delay in diagnosis resulted in long-term health consequences for many workers.

3. **Mid-20th Century: Improved Awareness and the Emergence of Environmental Health**
By the mid-20th century, several high-profile environmental health disasters, such as the Minamata mercury poisoning in Japan and widespread lead poisoning from gasoline, increased awareness of heavy metal toxicity. Diagnostic testing became more refined, and public health initiatives began to focus on reducing environmental exposure. However, chronic low-level exposure remained difficult to detect, and many individuals suffered long-term health consequences before the true cause of their symptoms was identified.

Case Example: In the 1960s, researchers studying children living near lead smelting plants found that even low-level lead exposure was linked to reduced IQ and developmental delays. This discovery led to the gradual removal of lead from gasoline and paints, dramatically reducing childhood lead poisoning in many countries.

4. **Present Day: Comprehensive Testing but Persistent Misdiagnosis**
Today, we have a broader range of diagnostic tools, including hair analysis, urine challenge tests, and advanced imaging techniques. Despite these advancements, heavy metal toxicity is still often missed or misdiagnosed due to non-specific

symptoms, limited awareness among healthcare providers, and the lack of routine screening for heavy metals. Patients with chronic symptoms may go through numerous misdiagnoses before the true cause is identified.

Case Example: A woman in her 30s suffered from chronic migraines, muscle weakness, and anxiety for several years. She visited multiple specialists and was diagnosed with conditions ranging from anxiety disorder to fibromyalgia. After extensive testing, she discovered elevated levels of mercury and arsenic, likely from years of consuming contaminated seafood and using herbal remedies containing arsenic. Once she underwent detoxification, her symptoms improved significantly, illustrating the value of comprehensive testing even in modern clinical practice.

Summary

Chapter 12 presents a collection of case studies that highlight the challenges and complexities of diagnosing heavy metal toxicity across different eras. The chapter illustrates how misdiagnosis and delayed diagnosis can lead to prolonged suffering and poor health outcomes. It also emphasises the need for increased awareness and comprehensive testing in modern clinical practice to avoid repeating the mistakes of the past.

By comparing diagnostic challenges across time periods, this chapter sheds light on how far we've come in understanding and diagnosing heavy metal toxicity and how much more needs to be done to ensure timely and accurate diagnoses for all patients. These lessons provide a foundation for exploring effective treatment protocols, which will be addressed in the following chapters.

.

Summary: Case Studies in Diagnosis

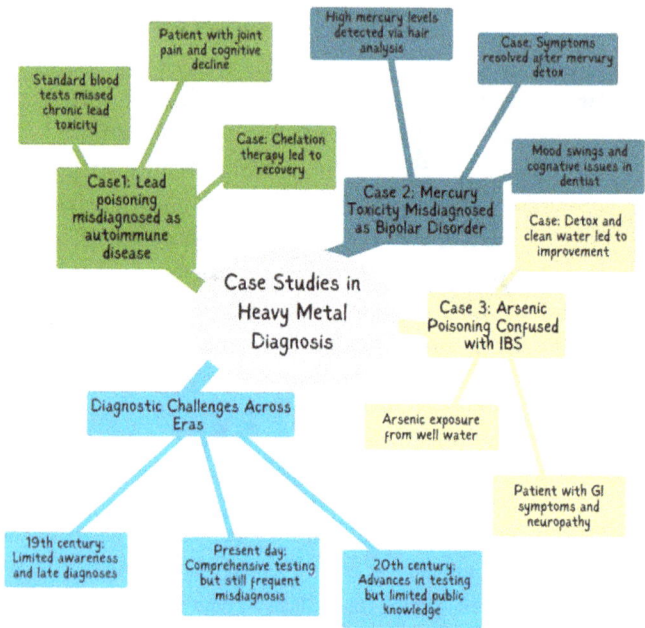

Patient with joint pain and cognitive decline

Standard blood tests missed chronic lead toxicity

High mercury levels detected via hair analysis

Case: Symptoms resolved after mercury detox

Case: Chelation therapy led to recovery

Case1: Lead poisoning misdiagnosed as autoimmune disease

Mood swings and cognative issues in dentist

Case 2: Mercury Toxicity Misdiagnosed as Bipolar Disorder

Case: Detox and clean water led to improvement

Case Studies in Heavy Metal Diagnosis

Case 3: Arsenic Poisoning Confused with IBS

Diagnostic Challenges Across Eras

Arsenic exposure from well water

Patient with GI symptoms and neuropathy

19th century: Limited awareness and late diagnoses

Present day: Comprehensive testing but still frequent misdiagnosis

20th century: Advances in testing but limited public knowledge

Chapter 13: Medical Interventions for Heavy Metal Toxicity

Chelation Therapy: Mechanisms, Risks, and Benefits

Chelation therapy is one of the primary medical interventions used to treat heavy metal toxicity. It involves the administration of chelating agents—substances that bind to heavy metals and facilitate their excretion from the body. While chelation can be highly effective, it also carries risks and potential side effects, making it essential for healthcare providers to carefully assess when and how to use this therapy.

1. **How Chelation Therapy Works**
   Chelating agents are compounds with a strong affinity for metal ions. When introduced into the body, they bind to heavy metals like lead, mercury, and arsenic, forming stable complexes that can be excreted through the urine or feces. The choice of chelating agent depends on the specific metal and the severity of the toxicity. Common chelating agents include:
   a. **Dimercaprol (BAL)**: Primarily used for acute arsenic, lead, or mercury poisoning. It is administered intramuscularly and is often combined with other chelating agents for enhanced efficacy.
   b. **Calcium Disodium EDTA**: Effective for lead toxicity. It is typically administered intravenously and can rapidly reduce blood lead levels. However, it may deplete essential minerals like calcium and zinc.
   c. **DMSA (Dimercaptosuccinic Acid)**: An oral chelator used for lead and mercury toxicity. It is considered safer and has fewer side effects compared to BAL.
   d. **DMPS (Dimercaptopropane Sulfonate)**: An oral or intravenous chelator used for mercury, arsenic, and lead

poisoning. It is particularly effective in mobilising metals stored in tissues.

Analogy: Chelation therapy acts like a "molecular claw" that grabs onto toxic metals and pulls them out of hiding, making them easier for the body to eliminate.

Case Study: Chelation Therapy for Severe Lead Poisoning

A 6-year-old child with dangerously high blood lead levels (over 45 mcg/dL) was treated with intravenous EDTA. After a five-day course of chelation therapy, his blood lead levels dropped significantly, and his symptoms of irritability and abdominal pain began to improve. However, the child also experienced mild side effects such as nausea and a transient drop in calcium levels, highlighting the need for careful monitoring during chelation therapy.

2. **Benefits of Chelation Therapy**
   a. **Rapid Reduction of Metal Burden:** Chelation therapy can quickly reduce the body's heavy metal burden, particularly in cases of acute poisoning. This rapid action is crucial for preventing permanent organ damage.
   b. **Symptom Relief and Health Improvement:** Chelation has been shown to alleviate symptoms such as fatigue, cognitive impairment, and neuropathy associated with heavy metal toxicity. Patients often report significant improvements in their quality of life after completing chelation therapy.
   c. **Prevention of Long-Term Complications:** By removing heavy metals from the body, chelation therapy can prevent long-term complications such as kidney damage, cardiovascular disease, and neurodegenerative conditions.

3. **Risks and Side Effects**
   While chelation therapy is generally effective, it is not without risks. Potential side effects include:

a. **Electrolyte Imbalance:** Chelating agents can bind to essential minerals like calcium, magnesium, and zinc, leading to imbalances that may cause muscle cramps, fatigue, and heart palpitations.

b. **Kidney Damage:** In rare cases, chelation therapy can overload the kidneys, leading to renal toxicity, especially in patients with pre-existing kidney conditions.

c. **Redistribution of Metals:** Improper use of chelating agents can result in the redistribution of metals to other tissues, potentially worsening symptoms.

Analogy: Chelation therapy is like "flushing out a clogged drain" — if not done carefully, it can cause the toxic sludge to spread elsewhere, making the problem worse instead of better.

Case Study: Complications of Chelation Therapy in a Patient with Pre-Existing Kidney Disease

A 55-year-old man with chronic kidney disease and a history of lead exposure underwent chelation therapy with EDTA. After the first session, he developed acute renal failure due to the additional burden placed on his kidneys. The therapy was discontinued, and the patient required hospitalisation for supportive care. This case highlights the need for careful patient selection and monitoring during chelation therapy, particularly in individuals with compromised kidney function.

4. **Guidelines for Safe Use of Chelation Therapy**
   To minimise risks, chelation therapy should be administered under the supervision of a healthcare professional with experience in managing heavy metal toxicity. Pre-treatment evaluation should include a thorough medical history, assessment of kidney function, and baseline levels of essential minerals. During therapy, regular monitoring of renal function, electrolyte levels, and metal excretion is essential to ensure safety and efficacy.

Analogy: Administering chelation therapy is like "walking a tightrope" — it requires careful balance and precision to achieve the desired outcome without causing harm.

Other Pharmaceutical Interventions

In addition to chelation therapy, other pharmaceutical interventions can be used to support detoxification and alleviate symptoms of heavy metal toxicity. These therapies are often used as adjuncts to chelation or in cases where chelation is not appropriate.

1. **Antioxidants**
   Heavy metals generate oxidative stress, which damages cells and tissues. Antioxidants such as vitamin C, vitamin E, glutathione, and N-acetylcysteine (NAC) can help neutralise free radicals and reduce oxidative damage. Glutathione, in particular, plays a crucial role in cellular detoxification and can be administered orally or intravenously to support the body's ability to eliminate heavy metals.

   Analogy: Antioxidants are like "fire extinguishers" that put out the oxidative stress fires started by heavy metals.

   Case Study: Intravenous Glutathione for Mercury Detoxification

   A 45-year-old woman with chronic mercury toxicity received intravenous glutathione therapy as part of her detoxification protocol. After a series of treatments, her symptoms of brain fog and fatigue improved significantly. This case demonstrates the supportive role of antioxidants in managing heavy metal toxicity

2. **Medications for Symptomatic Relief**
   a. **Chelation Adjuncts:** Drugs such as Penicillamine and Trientine are sometimes used as adjuncts to primary chelating agents for conditions like copper toxicity.
   b. **Symptom Management:** Medications may be used to manage symptoms such as pain, neuropathy, or

gastrointestinal disturbances in patients with heavy metal toxicity. For example, Gabapentin or Pregabalin may be prescribed to alleviate nerve pain associated with metal-induced neuropathy.

Analogy: These medications act like "buffers," providing relief from the symptoms caused by heavy metals while the body undergoes detoxification.

Combining Medical Interventions with Functional Approaches

While medical interventions like chelation and pharmaceutical support are effective for reducing heavy metal burden, combining these treatments with functional medicine approaches can enhance overall outcomes. Functional medicine focuses on supporting the body's natural detoxification pathways through nutrition, supplementation, and lifestyle modifications.

1. **Nutritional Support**

   A diet rich in antioxidants, fibre, and detox-supporting nutrients (e.g., sulphur-containing foods like garlic and cruciferous vegetables) can enhance the body's ability to eliminate heavy metals. Specific nutrients such as zinc, selenium, and magnesium help protect against the toxic effects of metals by competing for absorption and supporting enzymatic functions.

   Analogy: Nutritional support acts like "reinforcing the body's defences," providing it with the tools it needs to combat toxicity.

2. **Supplementation**
   Supplements such as chlorella, spirulina, and activated charcoal can bind to heavy metals in the digestive tract, reducing reabsorption and promoting elimination through the stool. Milk thistle and alpha-lipoic acid support liver function, enhancing the body's detoxification capacity.

Case Study: Chlorella Supplementation in a Patient with Mercury Toxicity

A 50-year-old man with elevated mercury levels added chlorella supplements to his chelation therapy. Over six months, his mercury levels gradually decreased, and his digestive health improved. Chlorella's ability to bind metals in the gut helped reduce reabsorption and facilitated more effective detoxification.

3. **Lifestyle Modifications**
    Avoiding known sources of heavy metal exposure (e.g., eliminating fish high in mercury or using air purifiers to reduce environmental pollutants) can prevent further accumulation of toxins during treatment. Regular exercise, adequate hydration, and stress management are also essential for supporting the body's detoxification processes.

    Analogy: Lifestyle modifications are like "locking the door" to prevent new toxins from entering the body while existing ones are being removed.

Summary

Chapter 13 provides an in-depth exploration of medical interventions for heavy metal toxicity, focusing on the mechanisms, benefits, and risks of chelation therapy. It also discusses other pharmaceutical options and the value of combining conventional treatments with functional medicine approaches. Through detailed case studies and vivid analogies, this chapter highlights the importance of individualised treatment plans and careful monitoring to achieve the best outcomes while minimising risks. The next chapter will delve deeper into functional medicine and alternative therapies for treating heavy metal toxicity, building on the foundational medical interventions discussed here.

Summary: Medical Interventions for Heavy Metal Toxicity

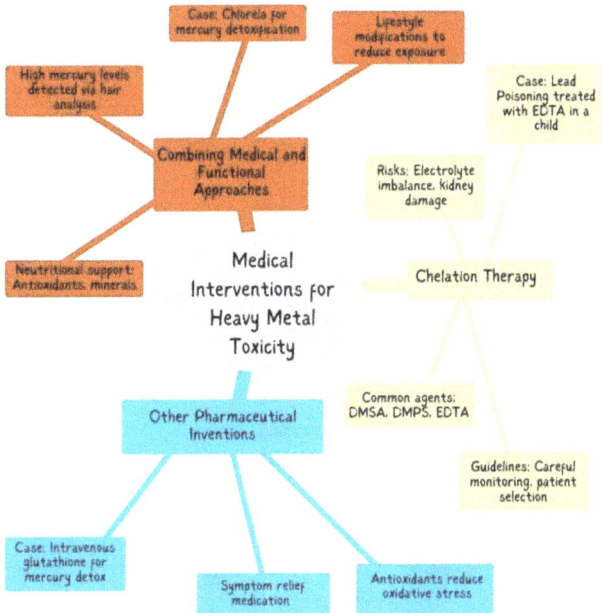

Medical Interventions for Heavy Metal Toxicity

Combining Medical and Functional Approaches
- Case: Chlorela for mercury detoxication
- Lifestyle modifications to reduce exposure
- High mercury levels detected via hair analysis
- Neutritional support: Antioxidants, minerals

Chelation Therapy
- Case: Lead Poisoning treated with EDTA in a child
- Risks: Electrolyte imbalance, kidney damage
- Common agents: DMSA, DMPS, EDTA
- Guidelines: Careful monitoring, patient selection

Other Pharmaceutical Inventions
- Case: Intravenous glutathione for mercury detox
- Symptom relief medication
- Antioxidants reduce oxidative stress

Chapter 14: Functional Medicine and Alternative Therapies for Heavy Metal Detoxification

Nutritional Support and Detox Protocols

Functional medicine approaches to heavy metal detoxification emphasise the importance of supporting the body's natural detox pathways through a combination of diet, nutritional supplements, and lifestyle modifications. These strategies aim to enhance the liver, kidneys, and gastrointestinal tract's ability to process and eliminate toxins, thereby reducing the overall toxic burden.

1. **Dietary Strategies for Detoxification**
   The foundation of any detox protocol is a diet that supports the body's natural elimination processes. A heavy metal detox diet typically includes:
   a. **High-Antioxidant Foods:** Antioxidants neutralise free radicals produced by heavy metal exposure. Foods rich in antioxidants, such as berries, dark leafy greens, and colourful vegetables, help protect cells from oxidative damage.
   b. **Sulphur-Rich Foods:** Sulphur-containing foods like garlic, onions, and cruciferous vegetables (e.g., broccoli, cabbage, Brussels sprouts) promote the production of glutathione, a powerful antioxidant and detoxifier that helps eliminate heavy metals.
   c. **Fibre-Rich Foods:** Fibre binds to heavy metals in the digestive tract, preventing reabsorption and promoting their excretion. Whole grains, legumes, and fruits provide ample fibre to support bowel regularity and toxin elimination.

Analogy: Think of these foods as "cleansing agents" for the body, helping to sweep away toxins and keep detox pathways clear.

Case Study: Dietary Changes in a Patient with Mercury Toxicity

A 50-year-old woman diagnosed with mercury toxicity switched to a high-antioxidant, sulphur-rich diet. Over a period of six months, she noticed improvements in her cognitive function, energy levels, and overall well-being. Laboratory tests showed a gradual reduction in mercury levels, supporting the efficacy of dietary interventions as part of a comprehensive detoxification plan.

2. **Supplementation for Enhanced Detoxification**
   Certain supplements can enhance the body's ability to detoxify heavy metals. Some of the most effective supplements for heavy metal detox include:
   a. **Chlorella and Spirulina:** These algae-based supplements have strong binding properties, allowing them to capture heavy metals in the digestive tract and promote their elimination through the stool.
   b. **N-Acetylcysteine (NAC) and Glutathione:** NAC is a precursor to glutathione, a key antioxidant that supports detoxification. Supplementing with NAC or glutathione can enhance the body's ability to neutralise and excrete heavy metals.
   c. **Activated Charcoal and Bentonite Clay:** These substances act as adsorbents, trapping heavy metals in the gut and preventing their reabsorption. They are particularly useful for managing gastrointestinal symptoms associated with heavy metal detox.

Analogy: Supplements like chlorella and activated charcoal are like "sponges" that soak up toxins, preventing them from being reabsorbed and causing further damage.

Case Study: Spirulina and Chlorella for Reducing Heavy Metal Levels

A 42-year-old man with elevated lead levels began taking a combination of spirulina and chlorella as part of his detox protocol. After three months of consistent use, his lead levels dropped significantly, and his energy and cognitive function improved. This case demonstrates the effectiveness of these supplements in reducing the body's heavy metal burden.

3. **Support for Liver and Kidney Function**
   The liver and kidneys play crucial roles in detoxification. Supporting these organs with specific nutrients can enhance their ability to process and eliminate heavy metals:
   a. **Milk Thistle:** Contains silymarin, which protects liver cells from oxidative damage and supports regeneration.
   b. **Dandelion Root:** Acts as a gentle diuretic, promoting kidney function and urine production, which facilitates the excretion of toxins.

Analogy: Supporting liver and kidney function is like "strengthening the filters" of the body, ensuring that they can efficiently remove heavy metals and other toxins.

Case Study: Milk Thistle and Dandelion Root for Liver Support in a Patient Undergoing Chelation Therapy

A 35-year-old man undergoing chelation therapy for lead toxicity experienced mild elevations in liver enzymes. His doctor recommended supplementing with milk thistle and dandelion root. After four weeks, his liver enzyme levels normalised, allowing him to continue chelation therapy without interruption. This case highlights the importance of organ support during detoxification.

Herbal Remedies and Natural Chelators

Herbal remedies have long been used in traditional medicine to support detoxification and promote overall health. Some herbs and natural chelators have demonstrated the ability to bind to heavy metals, enhance their excretion, or reduce the oxidative stress caused by metal toxicity.

1. **Cilantro and Parsley**

   Cilantro (coriander) and parsley are known for their ability to mobilise heavy metals from tissues. Cilantro, in particular, has been studied for its potential to enhance the excretion of lead, mercury, and aluminium. When combined with other natural chelators like chlorella, it may improve the overall effectiveness of detox protocols.

   Analogy: Cilantro acts like a "magnet" that pulls metals out of hiding, while chlorella captures them and ensures they are carried out of the body.

   Case Study: Cilantro and Chlorella for Mercury Detoxification

   A 40-year-old woman with a history of mercury exposure began taking cilantro and chlorella supplements. After several months, her urine mercury levels increased, indicating enhanced mobilisation and excretion of mercury. This combination helped alleviate her symptoms of brain fog and fatigue.

2. **Turmeric and Curcumin**

   Turmeric, and its active compound curcumin, have potent anti-inflammatory and antioxidant properties. Curcumin can reduce the oxidative damage caused by heavy metals and support the body's detoxification pathways. Studies have shown that curcumin can protect against cadmium- and arsenic-induced toxicity in animal models.

   Analogy: Curcumin is like a "firefighter" that extinguishes the inflammation and oxidative stress caused by heavy metals, protecting cells from further damage.

Case Study: Turmeric Supplementation for Arsenic Toxicity

A 55-year-old man with chronic arsenic exposure from drinking contaminated water added turmeric supplements to his detox regimen. After three months, he reported reduced joint pain and improved skin health. Blood tests showed lower markers of oxidative stress, supporting the role of curcumin in mitigating the effects of heavy metal toxicity.

3. **Garlic (Allium sativum)**
   Garlic contains sulphur compounds that support detoxification and have been shown to reduce the toxic effects of lead and mercury. Studies suggest that garlic may enhance the excretion of heavy metals through the urine and protect against oxidative damage.

   Analogy: Garlic is like "a bodyguard" that shields cells from the harmful effects of heavy metals while escorting them out of the body.

   ### Case Study: Garlic for Lead Toxicity in Industrial Workers

   A group of factory workers exposed to lead were given garlic supplements for 12 weeks. Compared to a control group, the workers taking garlic had lower blood lead levels and fewer symptoms of lead toxicity, such as headaches and irritability. This study demonstrates garlic's potential as a natural, supportive treatment for heavy metal exposure.

Integrative and Holistic Therapies

In addition to dietary and herbal approaches, several integrative therapies can support the detoxification process and improve overall health outcomes in individuals with heavy metal toxicity.

1. **Infrared Sauna Therapy**
   Infrared sauna therapy promotes sweating, which helps eliminate heavy metals from the skin. Sweating has been shown

to excrete metals such as arsenic, cadmium, lead, and mercury, making sauna therapy a valuable adjunct to traditional detox methods.

Analogy: Infrared sauna therapy is like "opening additional escape routes" for heavy metals to leave the body.

Case Study: Infrared Sauna Use in a Patient with Chronic Cadmium Toxicity

A 47-year-old man with elevated cadmium levels incorporated weekly infrared sauna sessions into his detox protocol. After three months, his cadmium levels dropped significantly, and his symptoms of joint pain and chronic fatigue improved. The combination of sauna therapy and dietary interventions contributed to his successful detoxification.

2. **Hyperbaric Oxygen Therapy (HBOT)**
   HBOT involves breathing pure oxygen in a pressurised environment, which increases oxygen delivery to tissues and enhances the body's ability to heal. Some studies suggest that HBOT may help reduce oxidative stress and inflammation caused by heavy metal toxicity.

Analogy: HBOT is like "turbocharging" the body's natural healing mechanisms, providing additional support during detoxification.

Case Study: HBOT for Neurological Recovery in a Patient with Mercury Toxicity

A 55-year-old woman with chronic mercury toxicity and neurological symptoms, including tremors and memory loss, underwent HBOT sessions twice a week. After 10 sessions, she reported improved cognitive function and reduced tremors. This case suggests that HBOT may support neurological recovery in patients with heavy metal-induced damage.

3. **Acupuncture and Traditional Chinese Medicine (TCM)**

Acupuncture and TCM have been used for centuries to support detoxification and restore balance to the body. Acupuncture may help reduce symptoms of heavy metal toxicity by promoting circulation, reducing inflammation, and supporting organ function.

Analogy: Acupuncture acts like "a traffic controller," directing energy flow and optimising organ function to support detoxification.

Case Study: Acupuncture for Symptom Relief in a Patient with Lead Toxicity

A 60-year-old woman with chronic lead toxicity experienced severe joint pain and insomnia. After weekly acupuncture sessions for three months, her pain levels decreased, and she reported improved sleep. The use of acupuncture provided symptomatic relief, complementing her overall detoxification strategy.

Summary

Chapter 14 explores the functional and alternative therapies available for managing heavy metal toxicity. From dietary strategies and nutritional supplements to herbal remedies and integrative therapies, this chapter presents a comprehensive approach to detoxification. Through detailed case studies and vivid analogies, it illustrates how these therapies can enhance the body's natural ability to eliminate toxins, reduce oxidative stress, and support overall health during the detox process.

The chapter emphasises the importance of combining these natural approaches with conventional medical treatments to achieve optimal outcomes in patients with heavy metal toxicity. The next chapter will delve into the role of intravenous therapies and their efficacy in heavy metal detoxification.

Summary: Functional Medicine and Alternative Therapies for Heavy Metal Detoxification

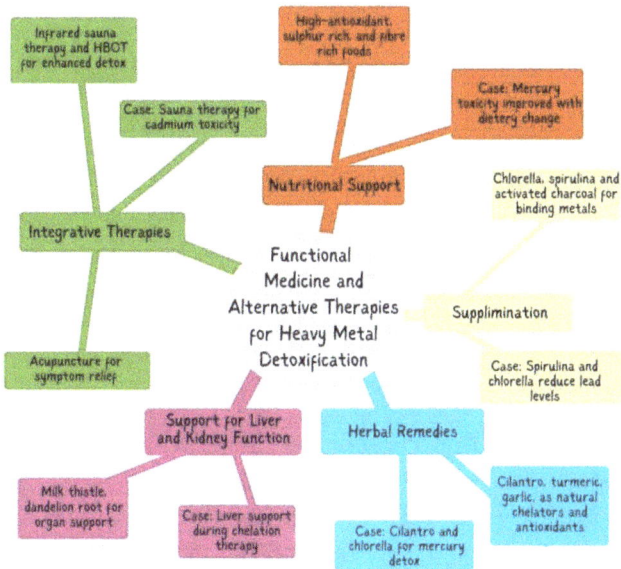

Functional Medicine and Alternative Therapies for Heavy Metal Detoxification

- Integrative Therapies
  - Infrared sauna therapy and HBOT for enhanced detox
  - Case: Sauna therapy for cadmium toxicity
  - Acupuncture for symptom relief
- Nutritional Support
  - High-antioxidant, sulphur rich and fibre rich foods
  - Case: Mercury toxicity improved with dietary change
- Supplimination
  - Chlorella, spirulina and activated charcoal for binding metals
  - Case: Spirulina and chlorella reduce lead levels
- Herbal Remedies
  - Cilantro, turmeric, garlic, as natural chelators and antioxidants
  - Case: Cilantro and chlorella for mercury detox
- Support for Liver and Kidney Function
  - Milk thistle, dandelion root for organ support
  - Case: Liver support during chelation therapy

Chapter 15: Intravenous Therapies for Heavy Metal Detoxification

Overview of Drip Therapies: Vitamin C, Glutathione, EDTA

Intravenous (IV) therapies are a cornerstone of integrative and functional medicine approaches for detoxifying the body from heavy metals. By delivering nutrients and chelating agents directly into the bloodstream, IV therapies bypass the digestive system, ensuring maximum absorption and effectiveness. This chapter will cover the most commonly used IV therapies, their mechanisms, benefits, and potential risks.

1. **Vitamin C Drip Therapy**
   High-dose vitamin C (ascorbic acid) is one of the most frequently used IV therapies in the treatment of heavy metal toxicity. Vitamin C is a powerful antioxidant that helps neutralise free radicals produced by heavy metals, thereby reducing oxidative stress. Additionally, vitamin C can chelate some heavy metals and promote their excretion through urine.
   Mechanism of Action: Vitamin C donates electrons to neutralise free radicals and supports glutathione production, an essential detoxifying agent in the liver. It can also bind to some metals like copper and promote their removal from the body.
   Benefits: Vitamin C IV therapy has been shown to improve energy levels, cognitive function, and overall health in patients with heavy metal toxicity. It also supports the immune system and helps reduce inflammation.
   Risks and Considerations: High-dose vitamin C can sometimes cause gastrointestinal discomfort, especially in patients with kidney issues or G6PD deficiency (a rare genetic condition that affects red blood cell function). Proper screening and monitoring are necessary to ensure safety.

Analogy: Vitamin C acts like a "fire extinguisher," quenching the flames of oxidative stress caused by heavy metals and supporting the body's detoxification pathways.

Case Study: Vitamin C Drip Therapy in a Patient with Arsenic Toxicity

A 45-year-old woman with chronic arsenic exposure received weekly high-dose vitamin C drips for three months. After the treatment, her energy levels and cognitive function improved significantly, and her urinary arsenic levels decreased by over 50%. The therapy reduced her oxidative stress and supported her overall health during the detoxification process.

2. **Glutathione Drip Therapy**

Glutathione is often referred to as the "master antioxidant" because of its crucial role in detoxification, immune function, and cellular health. IV glutathione therapy helps replenish depleted stores and supports the liver's ability to detoxify and eliminate heavy metals.

Mechanism of Action: Glutathione binds to metals such as mercury, lead, and cadmium, forming water-soluble complexes that can be excreted through bile or urine. It also enhances mitochondrial function and protects cells from oxidative damage.

Benefits: IV glutathione has been shown to reduce neurological symptoms, improve liver function, and enhance overall energy levels in patients with heavy metal toxicity.

Risks and Considerations: While generally safe, glutathione therapy may cause allergic reactions in rare cases. Additionally, it can temporarily mobilise metals into the bloodstream, which can exacerbate symptoms if not paired with adequate elimination support.

Analogy: Glutathione is like a "protective shield" that neutralises the toxic effects of heavy metals and supports the body's detoxification processes.

Case Study: Glutathione IV Therapy for Mercury Toxicity

A 50-year-old man with elevated mercury levels due to seafood consumption began weekly IV glutathione treatments. After three months, his cognitive symptoms, such as brain fog and memory loss, improved, and his mercury levels decreased significantly. This case highlights the efficacy of glutathione in reducing the toxic burden of mercury.

3. **EDTA Chelation Therapy**

Ethylenediaminetetraacetic acid (EDTA) is a synthetic amino acid used as a chelating agent to bind to heavy metals such as lead, cadmium, and arsenic. EDTA chelation therapy is typically administered intravenously and can quickly reduce blood levels of these metals.

Mechanism of Action: EDTA binds to metal ions, forming stable complexes that are then excreted through the urine. It is particularly effective for reducing lead and cadmium levels.

Benefits: EDTA chelation can prevent the long-term health effects of heavy metal exposure, such as cardiovascular disease, kidney damage, and cognitive decline. It has been shown to reduce symptoms like fatigue, joint pain, and neurological impairment.

Risks and Considerations: EDTA can deplete essential minerals such as calcium, magnesium, and zinc. It can also cause temporary side effects such as nausea, fatigue, and headache. Monitoring and supplementation with essential minerals are necessary during and after treatment.

Analogy: EDTA is like a "magnet" that pulls heavy metals out of hiding places and removes them from the body, but it must be used with care to avoid disrupting essential minerals.

Case Study: EDTA Chelation Therapy for Lead Exposure in an Industrial Worker

A 55-year-old industrial worker with elevated lead levels received bi-weekly EDTA chelation therapy for three months. His blood lead levels decreased significantly, and his symptoms of joint pain and fatigue improved. However, he experienced mild muscle cramps due to low calcium levels, which were corrected with supplementation.

Efficacy and Safety Concerns

While IV therapies can be highly effective for detoxifying the body, their use must be carefully managed to avoid potential complications. Several factors influence the efficacy and safety of IV therapies:

1. **Patient Selection and Pre-Treatment Evaluation**
   Not all patients are candidates for IV therapy. Individuals with certain medical conditions, such as kidney or liver disease, may not tolerate these treatments well. A thorough evaluation of kidney function, liver enzymes, and overall health status is essential before starting therapy.
   Analogy: Administering IV therapy without proper evaluation is like "setting off fireworks in a crowded room" — it can lead to unintended and dangerous outcomes.

2. **Dose and Frequency Management**

   The dosage and frequency of IV therapies must be tailored to the patient's needs and tolerance. Administering too high a dose too quickly can cause a rapid mobilisation of metals, leading to a worsening of symptoms or redistribution of metals to sensitive tissues. Gradual dosing and regular monitoring are crucial for ensuring safety and efficacy.
   Analogy: Managing IV therapy is like "turning a dial" — too high, and it becomes overwhelming; too low, and it may not be effective.

3. **Combination Therapies**
   IV therapies are often used in combination to maximise detoxification. For example, a patient may receive vitamin C, glutathione, and EDTA in separate sessions to target different aspects of heavy metal detoxification. Supporting therapies,

such as mineral supplementation and antioxidant support, are also used to prevent deficiencies and oxidative damage.

Analogy: Combining therapies is like "assembling a team" — each component has a specific role, and together they work synergistically to achieve the best outcome.

4. **Potential Side Effects and Complications**
   Side effects such as nausea, dizziness, and fatigue are relatively common but usually resolve quickly. More serious complications, such as kidney damage or mineral imbalances, are rare but can occur, particularly in vulnerable populations. Regular follow-up and blood testing are essential to detect and manage any adverse effects early.

   Analogy: Monitoring patients undergoing IV therapy is like "keeping a close eye on a simmering pot" — small changes can indicate larger problems and require immediate attention.

Case Histories of IV Therapy Success

Real-world case histories provide valuable insights into how IV therapies can be used to treat heavy metal toxicity effectively. The following examples illustrate the benefits and challenges of using IV therapies in clinical practice:

1. **Case History 1: Vitamin C and Glutathione IV Therapy for Lead Toxicity**
   Patient Profile: A 34-year-old woman with elevated blood lead levels (45 mcg/dL) and symptoms of fatigue, irritability, and difficulty concentrating.
   Treatment: The patient received weekly IV vitamin C and glutathione therapy for six weeks, along with dietary changes and oral supplements.
   Outcome: Her blood lead levels decreased to 15 mcg/dL, and her symptoms improved significantly. She reported increased energy, improved mood, and better cognitive function.
   Challenges: The patient experienced mild fatigue and nausea after the first two sessions, likely due to the mobilisation of lead.

Adjustments in dosing and additional hydration resolved these side effects.

Key Takeaway: This case highlights the importance of gradual dosing and patient monitoring during IV therapy to minimise side effects and achieve effective detoxification.

2. **Case History 2: EDTA Chelation for Severe Cadmium Toxicity in a Factory Worker**

   Patient Profile: A 50-year-old male factory worker with chronic exposure to cadmium. Symptoms included joint pain, muscle weakness, and hypertension. Blood tests showed elevated cadmium levels (10 times above normal).

   Treatment: He received bi-weekly EDTA chelation therapy for 12 weeks, along with intravenous magnesium and zinc to prevent depletion of essential minerals.

   Outcome: His cadmium levels decreased significantly, and his symptoms of joint pain and hypertension improved. He reported reduced muscle weakness and increased stamina.

   Challenges: The patient experienced transient headaches and muscle cramps, which were managed with mineral supplementation and adjustments to his treatment protocol.

   Key Takeaway: EDTA chelation, when combined with supportive therapies, can be highly effective for managing heavy metal toxicity in industrial workers.

3. **Case History 3: Combined IV Therapy for Mercury and Arsenic Toxicity in a Seafood Consumer**

   Patient Profile: A 55-year-old woman with a history of consuming large amounts of seafood presented with neurological symptoms such as tremors, memory loss, and anxiety. Lab tests revealed high levels of both mercury and arsenic.

   Treatment: The patient received a combination of IV glutathione, vitamin C, and EDTA chelation therapy over a period of three months. Supportive therapies included oral selenium and alpha-lipoic acid to enhance mercury excretion.

Outcome: Her mercury and arsenic levels dropped significantly, and her neurological symptoms improved. By the end of treatment, her tremors had resolved, and her cognitive function had returned to baseline.

Challenges: The patient experienced mild anxiety and fatigue during the initial stages of therapy, likely due to the mobilisation of metals. These symptoms resolved with adjustments in dosing and additional mineral support.

Key Takeaway: Combining IV therapies can be highly effective for managing multi-metal toxicity, but requires careful management and patient support.

Summary

Chapter 15 delves into the role of intravenous therapies in treating heavy metal toxicity, covering key therapies such as vitamin C, glutathione, and EDTA chelation. Through detailed explanations, real-world case studies, and vivid analogies, the chapter highlights the benefits and challenges of using IV therapies in clinical practice.

It emphasises the importance of individualised treatment plans, proper patient selection, and ongoing monitoring to ensure safety and efficacy. This chapter sets the stage for exploring how IV therapies can be integrated with other holistic approaches to create a comprehensive detoxification strategy, which will be discussed in the following chapters.

Summary: Intravenous Therapies for Heavy Metal Detoxification

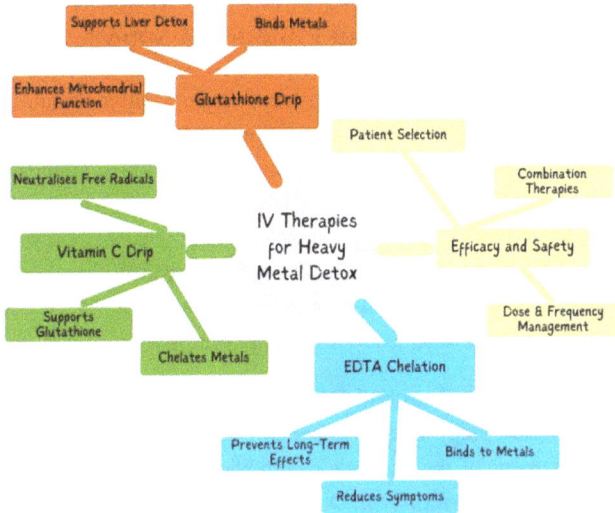

- Supports Liver Detox
- Binds Metals
- Enhances Mitochondrial Function
- Glutathione Drip
- Patient Selection
- Combination Therapies
- Neutralises Free Radicals
- Vitamin C Drip
- IV Therapies for Heavy Metal Detox
- Efficacy and Safety
- Supports Glutathione
- Chelates Metals
- Dose & Frequency Management
- EDTA Chelation
- Prevents Long-Term Effects
- Binds to Metals
- Reduces Symptoms

Chapter 16: General Treatment Protocols for Heavy Metal Detoxification

Combining Medical and Functional Approaches

Effective management of heavy metal toxicity often requires a multifaceted approach that combines conventional medical treatments with functional and holistic therapies. Integrating these methods provides a comprehensive strategy that addresses both the immediate removal of toxic metals and the long-term support of the body's detoxification pathways. This chapter will outline general treatment protocols that can be customised based on the patient's specific mental burden, health status, and symptoms.

1. **Initial Assessment and Diagnostic Testing**

   The first step in any treatment protocol is a thorough assessment of the patient's health status, history of exposure, and current symptoms. Diagnostic testing should include a combination of blood tests, urine challenge tests, hair analysis, or advanced diagnostic techniques such as Oligoscan or intracellular mineral analysis.

   Objective: To establish a baseline understanding of the patient's mental burden and identify potential deficiencies in essential minerals that may complicate treatment.

   Analogy: This initial assessment is like "mapping out the battlefield" — it provides crucial information for devising a strategic plan that targets the root cause of toxicity.

   Case Example: A 42-year-old man presenting with unexplained fatigue and memory loss underwent a comprehensive diagnostic work-up. Blood and urine tests revealed elevated mercury and cadmium levels, while hair analysis showed low levels of magnesium and zinc. These findings guided the development of a personalised detox protocol that included mineral supplementation, dietary changes, and chelation therapy.

2. **Phase 1: Preparation and Stabilisation**

Before initiating detoxification, it is essential to prepare the body to handle the increased burden of mobilised heavy metals. This phase focuses on supporting the liver, kidneys, and gastrointestinal tract to optimise detoxification pathways and prevent the reabsorption of metals.

Key Interventions:

a. **Liver Support:** Milk thistle, alpha-lipoic acid, and glutathione supplementation help the liver process and excrete toxins more efficiently.

b. **Kidney Support:** Dandelion root and adequate hydration promote healthy kidney function and urine production.

c. **Digestive Support:** Dietary fibre, chlorella, and probiotics reduce the reabsorption of metals in the gut and promote regular bowel movements.

Analogy: Preparation is like "priming a pump" — ensuring all pathways are clear and functional before turning on the flow of detoxification.

Case Example: A 50-year-old woman with high lead levels was started on a two-week pre-detox protocol that included milk thistle, magnesium, and dandelion tea. After this phase, she began chelation therapy with fewer side effects and a more stable detoxification process.

3. **Phase 2: Active Detoxification and Metal Removal**

The active detoxification phase involves the use of chelation therapy, IV nutrients, and natural chelators to remove heavy metals from the body. This phase is tailored to the patient's tolerance and response to treatment.

Key Interventions:

a. **Chelation Therapy:** EDTA, DMSA, or DMPS chelation based on the type and severity of metal toxicity.

b. **IV Nutrients:** High-dose vitamin C, glutathione, and trace minerals to support cellular health and reduce oxidative stress.

c. **Natural Chelators:** Chlorella, cilantro, and spirulina to bind metals in the gut and promote elimination.

Analogy: Active detoxification is like "sending out a clean-up crew" — targeting areas of the body where metals are stored and mobilising them for removal.

Case Example: A 38-year-old woman with a history of mercury exposure received bi-weekly chelation therapy with DMSA, along with daily chlorella supplements and weekly glutathione IVs. Over three months, her mercury levels dropped by 70%, and her neurological symptoms significantly improved.

4. **Phase 3: Rebuilding and Regeneration**
   Once the majority of heavy metals have been removed, the focus shifts to rebuilding and regenerating tissues that have been damaged by toxicity. This phase aims to restore optimal nutrient levels, support mitochondrial function, and reduce inflammation.
   Key Interventions:
   a. **Nutritional Repletion:** Supplementing with magnesium, zinc, selenium, and B vitamins to replenish deficiencies and support enzyme function.
   b. **Mitochondrial Support:** CoQ10, acetyl-L-carnitine, and PQQ (pyrroloquinoline quinone) to enhance cellular energy production.
   c. **Anti-Inflammatory Support:** Omega-3 fatty acids, curcumin, and resveratrol to reduce residual inflammation and promote healing.

Analogy: The rebuilding phase is like "repairing the damage after a storm" — replenishing what has been lost and strengthening the body for future resilience.

Case Example: A 60-year-old man who completed chelation therapy for lead toxicity underwent a three-month regeneration protocol. This included high-dose omega-3s, CoQ10, and magnesium supplementation. His energy levels, mood, and cognitive function improved significantly, and follow-up testing showed balanced nutrient levels and reduced oxidative stress markers.

5. **Ongoing Maintenance and Prevention**
   After completing active detoxification and regeneration, patients are encouraged to continue with maintenance strategies to prevent re-accumulation of heavy metals and support long-term health.
   Key Interventions:
   a. **Dietary Strategies:** Maintaining a diet rich in antioxidants and detox-supporting nutrients.
   b. **Periodic Testing:** Regular testing to monitor metal levels and overall health status.
   c. **Lifestyle Modifications:** Avoiding known sources of heavy metals, such as certain types of seafood, old plumbing, and occupational exposures.

   Analogy: Ongoing maintenance is like "establishing a long-term defence plan" to prevent future intrusions and protect health.

   Case Example: A 55-year-old man who completed a successful detoxification protocol continued with quarterly hair analysis and adopted a low-toxin diet. He remained symptom-free, and his metal levels stayed within a healthy range.

Tailoring Treatment to Individual Cases

Heavy metal detoxification protocols must be tailored to each individual's unique needs, considering factors such as the type of heavy metal, duration of exposure, overall health status, and individual tolerance to treatment. Customisation of protocols ensures that detoxification is safe, effective, and sustainable.

1. **Personalising Chelation Therapy**
   The choice of chelating agent, dosage, and frequency should be based on the specific metal burden and the patient's response. For example, a patient with severe lead toxicity may benefit from aggressive EDTA chelation, while a patient with low-level mercury exposure may only need oral DMSA combined with natural chelators.

2. **Addressing Co-Morbid Conditions**
   Patients with co-morbid conditions such as kidney disease, cardiovascular disease, or autoimmune disorders require additional consideration. Detoxification protocols must be adjusted to prevent exacerbation of these conditions and to support overall health.

3. **Supporting Emotional and Mental Health**
   Heavy metal toxicity can have profound effects on mental and emotional well-being. Incorporating therapies such as mindfulness, cognitive-behavioural therapy (CBT), or acupuncture can support mental health during detoxification.

   Analogy: Tailoring treatment is like "customising a suit" — each element must be carefully adjusted to fit the unique shape and needs of the individual.

Case Histories of Customised Detox Protocols

Real-world case histories demonstrate the importance of individualised treatment protocols and provide valuable insights into effective detoxification strategies.

1. **Case History 1: Customised Detox for Multi-Metal Toxicity in a Construction Worker**
   Patient Profile: A 40-year-old male construction worker with elevated levels of lead, cadmium, and arsenic due to long-term occupational exposure. Symptoms included chronic fatigue, muscle pain, and mood disturbances.
   Customised Protocol: The patient underwent bi-weekly IV chelation therapy with EDTA for lead and DMSA for cadmium

and arsenic. He also received weekly glutathione IVs and daily supplements of chlorella, milk thistle, and magnesium.

Outcome: After four months, his heavy metal levels dropped significantly, and his symptoms improved. Follow-up testing showed a balanced mineral profile, indicating successful detoxification without depletion of essential nutrients.

Key Takeaway: A combination of chelating agents, IV nutrients, and natural chelators effectively managed multi-metal toxicity in this patient, demonstrating the value of a tailored approach.

2. **Case History 2: Gentle Detoxification for a Sensitive Patient with Mercury Toxicity**

   Patient Profile: A 55-year-old woman with high mercury levels and sensitivity to chelation agents. Symptoms included severe brain fog, anxiety, and chronic headaches.

   Customised Protocol: Due to her sensitivity, the patient received a gentle protocol with low-dose oral DMSA, weekly IV glutathione, and daily supplements of cilantro, spirulina, and selenium. She also engaged in infrared sauna therapy twice a week to support gentle detoxification.

   Outcome: Over six months, her mercury levels decreased, and her symptoms gradually improved. She tolerated the protocol well, with no major side effects.

   Key Takeaway: This case illustrates the importance of adjusting dosages and using supportive therapies for patients with sensitivities to standard chelation protocols.

3. **Case History 3: Rapid Detoxification for Acute Lead Poisoning in a Child**

   Patient Profile: A 5-year-old boy with acute lead poisoning (blood lead level >70 mcg/dL) due to ingestion of lead-based paint chips.

   Customised Protocol: The child received intensive IV EDTA chelation therapy under hospital supervision, along with mineral supplementation and dietary modifications to enhance detoxification.

Outcome: His blood lead levels dropped rapidly to a safe range within three weeks. The child's cognitive function and behaviour improved significantly.

Key Takeaway: Rapid intervention with IV chelation is crucial in acute cases to prevent long-term neurological damage, especially in children.

Summary

Chapter 16 provides a comprehensive overview of general treatment protocols for heavy metal detoxification, emphasising the integration of medical, functional, and holistic approaches. By presenting detailed case histories and tailored strategies, the chapter highlights the importance of individualised treatment plans to achieve safe and effective detoxification.

Through vivid analogies and real-world examples, the chapter illustrates how each phase of detoxification—preparation, active detox, regeneration, and maintenance—plays a critical role in supporting patients on their journey to recovery. The next chapter will explore global perspectives on heavy metal exposure and policy initiatives, providing a broader context for understanding the challenges of managing heavy metal toxicity on a global scale.

Summary: General Treatment Protocols for Heavy Metal Detoxification

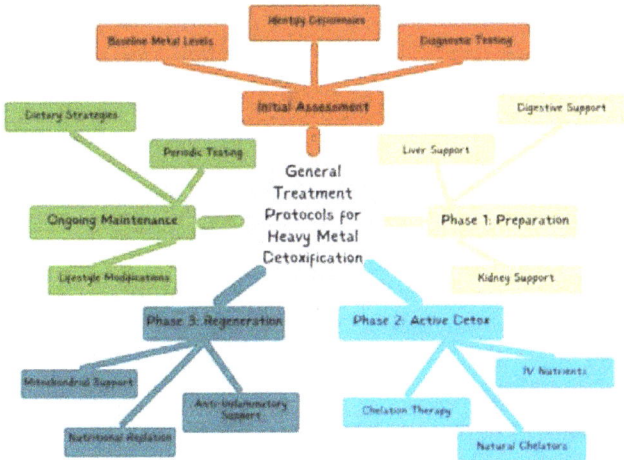

Chapter 17: Case Histories of Heavy Metal Toxicity Across Different Eras

Early 20th Century: Occupational Exposure and Industrialisation

The early 20th century marked a period of rapid industrialisation and urbanisation, bringing with it a surge in occupational exposure to heavy metals. Workers in industries such as mining, battery manufacturing, and chemical production were often exposed to hazardous levels of metals like lead, mercury, cadmium, and arsenic. At the time, the health impacts of these exposures were poorly understood, and safety regulations were minimal or non-existent. This chapter explores several historical case histories that highlight the challenges and health consequences faced by workers during this era.

1. **Case Study: Lead Poisoning in Battery Factory Workers**
    Location and Timeframe: United States, 1920s
    Background: During the early 1920s, the rapid growth of the automotive industry led to an increased demand for lead-acid batteries. Workers in battery factories were frequently exposed to lead dust and fumes without adequate protective equipment. Many experienced symptoms of lead poisoning, such as abdominal pain, muscle weakness, and severe fatigue.
    Health Impact: A study conducted in 1924 revealed that over 75% of workers in a major battery manufacturing plant had elevated blood lead levels and exhibited symptoms of lead toxicity. Chronic exposure led to long-term health issues, including kidney damage, neurological impairments, and increased mortality.
    Outcome: Public outcry and advocacy from labour unions led to the implementation of basic safety measures, such as improved ventilation and the use of personal protective

equipment (PPE). These changes marked the beginning of workplace health regulations, though enforcement remained inconsistent.

Analogy: The situation in battery factories during the early 20th century was like "working in a toxic fog" — employees were surrounded by invisible hazards that slowly but steadily eroded their health.

2. **Case Study: Mercury Exposure in Hatmakers ("Mad Hatter's Disease")**
   Location and Timeframe: England and the United States, early 1900s
   Background: Mercury nitrate was commonly used in the felting process to produce hats. Hatmakers were exposed to mercury vapours, which led to neurological symptoms such as tremors, memory loss, and mood disturbances — a condition colloquially known as "Mad Hatter's disease."
   Health Impact: Many hatmakers suffered from severe neurological impairments that were irreversible. The toxicity of mercury was not widely recognised, and affected workers were often dismissed as "insane" or suffering from personal problems.
   Outcome: It wasn't until the mid-20th century that mercury's role in these symptoms was scientifically established. As awareness grew, the use of mercury in the hat-making industry was phased out, and safer alternatives were adopted. This case history played a pivotal role in increasing public awareness of occupational hazards.

Analogy: The mercury exposure faced by hatmakers was like "a slow poisoning" — the symptoms were insidious and progressed over time, ultimately destroying the health and lives of many workers.

3. **Case Study: Arsenic Poisoning in Agricultural Workers**
Location and Timeframe: United States, 1930s
Background: Arsenic-based pesticides were widely used in the early 20th century to control insect populations in crops like cotton and fruit trees. Agricultural workers were often exposed to high levels of arsenic through inhalation and dermal absorption, resulting in a range of health issues.
Health Impact: Many workers developed symptoms of chronic arsenic poisoning, including skin lesions, respiratory problems, and gastrointestinal disturbances. Long-term exposure was linked to an increased risk of skin, lung, and bladder cancers.
Outcome: The health impacts of arsenic exposure were not widely recognised until the 1940s, when epidemiological studies linked arsenic use in agriculture to cancer rates in exposed populations. This led to stricter regulations on arsenic-based pesticides and, eventually, the development of safer alternatives.

Analogy: Working with arsenic-based pesticides was like "walking through a field of invisible landmines" — the risks were present but not immediately apparent, causing slow but devastating health consequences.

Mid-20th Century: Environmental Contaminations and Public Health Disasters

The mid-20th century saw several high-profile cases of environmental heavy metal contamination that had widespread health implications. These incidents raised public awareness about the dangers of heavy metal exposure and prompted changes in environmental policies and regulations.

1. **Case Study: Minamata Disease – Mercury Poisoning in Japan**
Location and Timeframe: Minamata Bay, Japan, 1950s-1960s
Background: The Chisso Corporation, a chemical manufacturer, discharged mercury-containing wastewater into

Minamata Bay for over three decades. This resulted in the accumulation of methylmercury in fish and shellfish, which were a primary food source for local residents.

Health Impact: Residents who consumed contaminated seafood developed severe neurological symptoms, including numbness, tremors, muscle weakness, and cognitive impairments. Children born to affected mothers exhibited congenital abnormalities and developmental delays. Hundreds of people died, and thousands more were affected.

Outcome: The Japanese government initially denied the connection between industrial pollution and health effects, leading to years of suffering for the local population. It wasn't until 1968 that the government officially recognised Minamata disease as mercury poisoning. Legal battles ensued, resulting in compensation for victims and stricter regulations on industrial waste disposal. The Minamata case became a global symbol of industrial pollution's impact on human health.

Analogy: The Minamata disaster was like "a silent tsunami" — it swept through the community, leaving devastation in its wake, but remained hidden beneath the surface for years.

2. **Case Study: Leaded Gasoline – A Global Public Health Crisis**
   Location and Timeframe: United States and Europe, 1920s-1980s
   Background: Lead was added to gasoline in the early 20th century to improve engine performance. The combustion of leaded gasoline released lead particles into the air, contaminating soil and water and exposing the population to lead.
   Health Impact: Lead exposure, particularly in children, was linked to lower IQ, developmental delays, behavioural problems, and increased risk of hypertension and kidney damage in adults. Entire generations suffered the consequences of widespread lead exposure.

Outcome: The harmful effects of leaded gasoline were documented as early as the 1920s, but it wasn't until the 1970s and 1980s that countries like the United States and those in Europe began phasing out leaded gasoline. The removal of lead from gasoline led to a dramatic decrease in blood lead levels and a significant public health victory.

Analogy: The impact of leaded gasoline on public health was like "a slow-burning fire" — it smouldered for decades, causing damage and loss of potential that wasn't fully recognised until it was almost too late.

3. **Case Study: Cadmium Contamination in Toyama, Japan ("Itai-Itai Disease")**
   Location and Timeframe: Toyama Prefecture, Japan, 1912-1960s
   Background: Mining operations released cadmium into the Jinzu River, contaminating the water used for irrigation. Local residents who consumed rice grown with contaminated water developed severe skeletal and kidney damage, a condition known as "Itai-Itai" disease (literally "It hurts, it hurts" disease).
   Health Impact: Patients experienced debilitating pain in their bones and joints, fractures, and renal dysfunction. The disease primarily affected older women, whose bones were already weakened by age and nutritional deficiencies.
   Outcome: After decades of suffering, the Japanese government finally recognised cadmium pollution as the cause of Itai-Itai disease in the 1960s. The mining company was held accountable, and victims were compensated. The case led to improved environmental regulations and awareness of industrial pollution's health effects.

   Analogy: The cadmium contamination in Toyama Prefecture was like "poison seeping into a well" — it tainted the lifeblood of the community, slowly crippling those who relied on it.

21st Century: Chronic Low-Level Exposure and Modern Health Impacts

In the 21st century, heavy metal exposure continues to be a significant public health concern, but the nature of exposure has shifted. Instead of acute or occupational exposure, most people are now exposed to low levels of heavy metals through environmental sources, consumer products, and contaminated food. Chronic low-level exposure can lead to subtle but significant health impacts that are often difficult to diagnose and attribute to heavy metal toxicity.

1. **Case Study: Chronic Mercury Exposure from Seafood Consumption**
   Location and Timeframe: United States, 2000s-Present
   Background: A 55-year-old woman with a history of high seafood consumption developed symptoms of chronic fatigue, brain fog, and peripheral neuropathy. Despite visiting numerous specialists, she was misdiagnosed with fibromyalgia and chronic fatigue syndrome. After several years, a comprehensive heavy metal test revealed elevated mercury levels, likely from regular consumption of large predatory fish such as tuna and swordfish.
   Health Impact: Chronic low-level mercury exposure led to neurological and cognitive impairment, which could have been prevented with early detection and dietary modifications.
   Outcome: The patient underwent a detoxification protocol that included IV glutathione and oral chelation therapy. Her symptoms improved over several months, and she adopted a diet that minimised her mercury exposure.
   Analogy: Chronic low-level mercury exposure is like "a slow leak in a dam" — it causes cumulative damage that can lead to a breakdown if not addressed in time.

2. **Case Study: Arsenic Contamination in Drinking Water in Bangladesh**
   Location and Timeframe: Bangladesh, 1990s-Present

Background: Millions of people in rural Bangladesh rely on groundwater for drinking water. Unfortunately, many of these water sources are contaminated with arsenic due to natural geological processes. Long-term consumption of arsenic-contaminated water has led to a public health crisis, with widespread cases of skin lesions, respiratory issues, and cancer.

Health Impact: Chronic arsenic exposure has been linked to high rates of skin, bladder, and lung cancers, as well as cardiovascular disease and diabetes. The crisis has affected generations of people and poses ongoing challenges for public health efforts.

Outcome: Despite international aid and public health campaigns, many people in rural areas continue to be exposed to dangerous levels of arsenic. Efforts to provide safe drinking water are ongoing, but progress has been slow due to economic and logistical barriers.

Analogy: The arsenic contamination in Bangladesh is like "a poisoned well" that keeps harming those who depend on it, generation after generation.

Summary

Chapter 17 provides a historical and global perspective on heavy metal toxicity through detailed case histories across different eras. From the occupational hazards of the early 20th century to environmental disasters of the mid-20th century and the chronic low-level exposures of the modern era, these stories illustrate the diverse ways in which heavy metals have impacted human health.

By comparing and contrasting the health impacts of heavy metal exposure across time and regions, this chapter underscores the ongoing challenge of managing heavy metal toxicity and highlights the need for continued vigilance, research, and policy initiatives. This comprehensive view sets the stage for discussing global distribution, policy implications, and environmental justice in the following chapter.

Summary: Case Histories of Heavy Metal Toxicity Across Different Eras

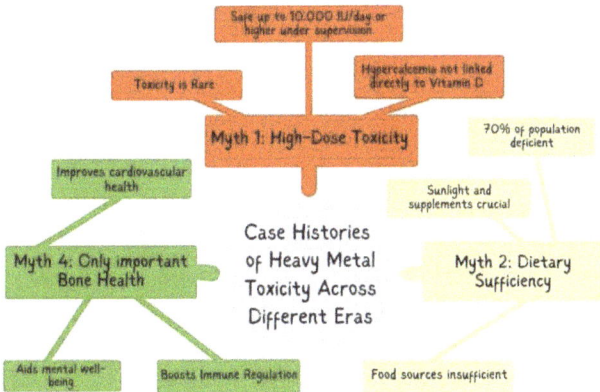

Chapter 18: Global Distribution of Heavy Metals and Environmental Justice

Geographic Variations in Heavy Metal Exposure

Heavy metal contamination varies significantly across different regions of the world due to a range of factors, including industrial activities, agricultural practices, and natural geological processes. While some areas have been able to mitigate exposure through stringent regulations and environmental policies, other regions—particularly in developing countries—continue to face high levels of contamination and health impacts. Understanding the global distribution of heavy metals is crucial for developing targeted interventions and policies that address this pervasive issue.

1. **Heavy Metals in Developed Nations**
   In developed nations such as the United States, Canada, and countries in the European Union, heavy metal exposure has generally decreased over the past few decades due to the implementation of environmental regulations and public health campaigns. For example, the removal of lead from gasoline and paint has significantly reduced lead exposure in children, and regulations on mercury emissions have curbed environmental contamination. However, certain populations within these nations, such as urban communities living near industrial sites or individuals consuming large amounts of seafood, continue to be at risk.

   Case Study: Lead Exposure in Low-Income Urban Communities in the United States

   Despite overall reductions in lead exposure, low-income communities in older urban areas continue to suffer from elevated blood lead levels due to ageing infrastructure and deteriorating lead-based paint in homes. A study conducted in 2016 found that children in low-income neighbourhoods of cities like Baltimore, Cleveland, and Chicago were up to five times more likely to have elevated blood lead levels compared to children in wealthier neighbourhoods. This ongoing disparity highlights the need for targeted interventions and policies that address environmental injustices within developed nations.

Analogy: The persistence of lead exposure in low-income urban areas is like "an invisible chain" that keeps pulling these communities back into a cycle of poor health and economic hardship.

2. **Heavy Metals in Developing Nations**
   Developing nations, particularly those undergoing rapid industrialisation such as China, India, and parts of Southeast Asia, face significant challenges with heavy metal contamination. Industrial activities such as mining, smelting, and manufacturing contribute to widespread contamination of air, soil, and water. Additionally, the use of heavy metal-based pesticides and fertilisers in agriculture increases the risk of exposure for both agricultural workers and consumers.

Case Study: Cadmium and Arsenic Contamination in China's "Cancer Villages"

In rural areas of China, high levels of cadmium and arsenic have been detected in soil and water, leading to the emergence of "cancer villages"—communities with unusually high rates of cancer. The contamination is often linked to nearby mining or smelting operations, which release toxic metals into the environment. Residents of these villages have reported increased incidences of lung, liver, and bladder cancers. Despite efforts by the Chinese government to regulate industrial emissions, enforcement remains inconsistent, and affected communities often lack the resources to relocate or access clean water sources.

Analogy: The situation in China's cancer villages is like "a slow poison seeping into the roots" of these communities, causing long-term harm that may not be fully realised for generations.

3. **Heavy Metals in Agriculture and Food Supply**
Heavy metal contamination is not limited to industrial activities. The widespread use of arsenic-based pesticides, lead-contaminated irrigation water, and cadmium-rich fertilisers can lead to contamination of crops and livestock, introducing toxic metals into the food chain. This is a particular concern in countries with poor agricultural regulations and oversight, where contaminated food products may be consumed domestically or exported, potentially affecting populations far beyond the point of origin.

Case Study: Arsenic in Rice from South Asia

Arsenic contamination of groundwater in countries such as Bangladesh, India, and Pakistan has led to high levels of arsenic in rice, a staple food in these regions. Chronic consumption of arsenic-contaminated rice has been linked to skin lesions, respiratory issues, and an increased risk of cancer. The problem is exacerbated by the fact that many rural communities rely on contaminated groundwater for irrigation, making it difficult to produce safe crops without significant investment in alternative water sources or crop management practices.

Analogy: The contamination of rice in South Asia is like "a poisoned staple" — a basic food source that nourishes millions but simultaneously exposes them to health risks.

Impact of Industrialisation in Developing Countries

As developing nations undergo rapid Industrialisation, the drive for economic growth often comes at the expense of environmental health and safety. Lax regulations, lack of enforcement, and the prioritisation of economic gain over environmental protection have resulted in widespread heavy metal contamination. The long-term health impacts of this contamination are often borne disproportionately by the poorest and most vulnerable populations, raising issues of environmental justice and equity.

1. **Mining and Smelting Operations**
   Mining and smelting are major sources of heavy metal contamination in developing countries. For example, artisanal gold mining in sub-Saharan Africa and South America often involves the use of mercury to extract gold from ore, resulting in significant mercury pollution of local water sources. Similarly, unregulated mining operations in countries such as Zambia and the Democratic Republic of Congo have led to elevated levels of lead, cadmium, and other metals in nearby communities. Residents suffer from high rates of kidney disease, neurological disorders, and developmental delays in children.

Case Study: Lead Poisoning in Kabwe, Zambia

Kabwe, once known as the "lead capital of Africa," has one of the highest levels of lead contamination in the world due to decades of lead mining and smelting. Despite the closure of the mine in 1994, residents, particularly children, continue to suffer from severe lead poisoning. A study conducted in 2017 found that over 90% of children tested had blood lead levels exceeding international safety limits. Efforts to remediate the environment have been slow, and the community remains trapped in a cycle of poverty and poor health.

Analogy: The situation in Kabwe is like "a toxic legacy" — the contamination persists long after the mine's closure, continuing to affect new generations.

2. **E-Waste Recycling and Heavy Metal Exposure**
   The global demand for electronic devices has led to the rise of e-waste recycling industries in countries like Ghana, Nigeria, and India. Informal recycling operations often involve burning or acid leaching of electronic components, releasing heavy metals such as lead, cadmium, and mercury into the

environment. Workers, including children, are directly exposed to toxic fumes and dust, resulting in high rates of respiratory issues, skin disorders, and neurological symptoms.

Case Study: E-Waste Recycling in Agbogbloshie, Ghana

Agbogbloshie, known as one of the world's largest e-waste dumpsites, is home to a thriving informal recycling industry. Workers, many of whom are teenagers, extract metals from discarded electronics with little to no protective equipment. Studies have found that blood lead levels in children living in Agbogbloshie are up to 20 times higher than in children living in uncontaminated areas. The community suffers from widespread health issues, but economic necessity drives many to continue working in hazardous conditions.

Analogy: The e-waste recycling industry in Agbogbloshie is like "a double-edged sword" — it provides economic opportunities while simultaneously posing severe health risks.

Environmental Justice and Policy Implications

Environmental justice refers to the fair treatment and meaningful involvement of all people, regardless of race, colour, national origin, or income, in the development, implementation, and enforcement of environmental laws, regulations, and policies. Unfortunately, when it comes to heavy metal contamination, marginalised and low-income communities around the world are disproportionately affected. These communities often lack the resources, political power, and social capital to advocate for cleaner environments and better health outcomes.

1. **Disproportionate Burden on Vulnerable Populations**
    Vulnerable populations, including indigenous communities, low-income families, and residents of Industrialised regions, are more likely to experience the harmful effects of heavy metal exposure. These groups are often situated near sources of contamination, such as mines, factories, or waste disposal sites,

and have limited access to healthcare and legal resources. For example, Native American communities in the United States have been disproportionately affected by uranium mining, while indigenous populations in the Amazon basin have suffered from mercury contamination due to illegal gold mining.

Case Study: Mercury Poisoning in the Amazon Basin

Illegal gold mining in the Amazon basin has led to significant mercury contamination of rivers and fish, a primary food source for indigenous communities. Mercury exposure has resulted in neurological impairments, developmental delays in children, and increased rates of miscarriage and stillbirths. Despite these severe health impacts, political and economic interests have hindered effective regulation and enforcement, leaving indigenous populations at the mercy of ongoing contamination.

Analogy: The mercury contamination in the Amazon is like "a spreading stain" that seeps into every aspect of life, leaving few places untouched.

2. **Policy Implications and Global Initiatives**

Addressing the global distribution of heavy metals requires coordinated efforts at both the national and international levels. Initiatives such as the Minamata Convention on Mercury, which seeks to reduce mercury emissions and protect vulnerable populations, are steps in the right direction. However, enforcement remains a challenge, particularly in countries with weak regulatory frameworks and limited resources.

Case Study: Minamata Convention on Mercury

The Minamata Convention, adopted in 2013, is a global treaty aimed at protecting human health and the environment from anthropogenic emissions and releases of mercury. While it has led to increased awareness and some reductions in mercury use, its impact has been limited by non-compliance and lack of funding for enforcement in low-income countries.

Analogy: The Minamata Convention is like "a shield with gaps" — it provides some protection but leaves many vulnerable to ongoing harm.

Summary

Chapter 18 explores the global distribution of heavy metals, highlighting geographic variations, the impact of industrialisation, and the disproportionate burden on vulnerable populations. Through detailed case studies and vivid analogies, the chapter illustrates how heavy metal contamination is not only an environmental issue but also a matter of environmental justice.

The chapter calls for stronger international cooperation and policy enforcement to address these disparities and protect at-risk communities. This sets the stage for discussing the role of heavy metals in dentistry, another important yet often overlooked source of exposure, which will be covered in the following chapter.

Summary: Global Distribution of Heavy Metals and Environmental Justice

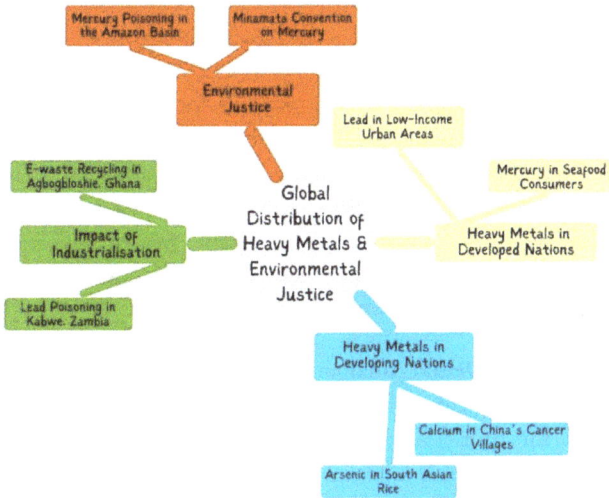

Chapter 19: Heavy Metals in Dentistry – A Hidden Health Risk

The Use of Heavy Metals in Dental Practices

Dentistry has long been a source of heavy metal exposure, with materials such as mercury, lead, and nickel being commonly used in dental amalgams, orthodontic appliances, and crowns. While advances in dental materials have reduced the use of some toxic metals, millions of people still have dental work that contains these elements, raising concerns about chronic exposure and potential health impacts.

1. **Mercury in Dental Amalgams**

   Dental amalgams, also known as "silver fillings," have been used for over 150 years to restore decayed teeth. These amalgams typically contain about 50% elemental mercury, along with other metals such as silver, tin, and copper. Mercury in amalgams is released as vapour, which can be inhaled or absorbed through the oral mucosa.

   Health Impact: Chronic exposure to mercury from dental amalgams has been associated with a variety of health issues, including neurological symptoms (e.g., memory loss, tremors, and anxiety), immune dysfunction, and kidney damage. While the American Dental Association (ADA) maintains that amalgams are safe, many countries have restricted their use, especially in vulnerable populations such as pregnant women and children.

   Case Study: Neurological Symptoms Linked to Dental Amalgams

   A 45-year-old woman with 10 amalgam fillings began experiencing chronic headaches, fatigue, and difficulty concentrating. Her mercury levels were found to be elevated.

After a safe amalgam removal procedure, her symptoms gradually improved over the course of six months. This case highlights the potential for chronic mercury exposure from amalgams to contribute to neurological symptoms.

Analogy: Dental amalgams are like "ticking time bombs" — they release small amounts of mercury over time, which can accumulate in the body and potentially cause health issues.

2. **Nickel in Orthodontic Appliances and Crowns**
Nickel is a common metal used in orthodontic appliances such as braces and in crowns or bridges made from metal alloys. While nickel is not as toxic as some other heavy metals, it is a known allergen and can cause contact dermatitis and systemic allergic reactions in sensitive individuals.
Health Impact: Prolonged exposure to nickel through dental appliances can lead to allergic reactions, which may manifest as oral ulcers, gingival inflammation, or skin rashes. In rare cases, systemic symptoms such as headaches, fatigue, and joint pain have been reported.

Case Study: Nickel Allergy in a Patient with Orthodontic Braces
A 16-year-old girl developed persistent mouth ulcers and gingival swelling after getting orthodontic braces. Patch testing confirmed a nickel allergy. The braces were replaced with nickel-free alternatives, and her symptoms resolved within weeks.

Analogy: Nickel in dental appliances is like "an irritant under the skin" — it can cause a range of symptoms in those with sensitivities, affecting their quality of life.

3. **Lead in Dental Crowns and Other Restorations**
Some dental crowns and restorations made with metal alloys may contain trace amounts of lead. Lead exposure from dental restorations is generally low, but it can add to the cumulative

burden of lead in individuals already exposed through other sources, such as contaminated water or soil.

Health Impact: While the health risks from lead in dental materials are not well-studied, any additional lead exposure is of concern, particularly in children and pregnant women, due to its neurotoxic effects.

Case Study: Elevated Blood Lead Levels in a Child with Metal Crowns

A 7-year-old boy with metal crowns had elevated blood lead levels despite no known environmental exposure. Analysis of the dental crowns revealed trace amounts of lead. After the crowns were replaced with ceramic alternatives, his blood lead levels decreased.

Analogy: The presence of lead in dental materials is like "a hidden trap" — it's not immediately obvious but can contribute to long-term health risks.

Health Risks and Controversies

The health risks associated with heavy metals in dental materials remain a topic of debate. While professional dental organisations such as the ADA and the World Health Organisation (WHO) maintain that dental amalgams and other metal-based materials are generally safe, growing evidence suggests that certain individuals may be more susceptible to adverse health effects. This section explores some of the key controversies and current scientific understanding.

1. **The Mercury Debate: Safe or Dangerous?**
   The safety of mercury in dental amalgams is one of the most contentious issues in modern dentistry. Proponents argue that the amount of mercury released from amalgams is too small to pose a significant health risk and that amalgams provide a durable, cost-effective solution for dental restorations. However, critics point to studies showing that even low levels of mercury exposure can have negative health effects,

particularly on the nervous system and immune function. Some countries, including Sweden, Norway, and Denmark, have banned the use of dental amalgams altogether, citing health and environmental concerns.

Case Study: Cognitive Decline and Chronic Fatigue Reversed After Amalgam Removal

A 55-year-old man with 12 amalgam fillings experienced cognitive decline, chronic fatigue, and irritability for several years. Despite undergoing numerous tests, no clear diagnosis was made. After his dentist recommended the safe removal of his amalgam fillings, his symptoms gradually improved over the next year. His experience underscores the need for a personalised approach to dental material safety.

Analogy: The debate over mercury in dental amalgams is like "a double-edged sword" — the same material that restores a tooth can potentially harm other parts of the body.

2. **Emerging Concerns: Bioaccumulation and Genetic Susceptibility**
   Recent research suggests that individuals with certain genetic predispositions, such as those with polymorphisms in the glutathione pathway, may be more vulnerable to the toxic effects of mercury and other metals. These individuals may have a reduced ability to detoxify and eliminate metals, leading to bioaccumulation and chronic health issues. This finding has led to calls for more personalised approaches to dental material selection, particularly in patients with a history of metal sensitivities or chronic health conditions.

Analogy: The concept of genetic susceptibility is like "a key that unlocks hidden vulnerabilities" — for some, the presence of heavy metals can open the door to a range of health problems.

3. **Environmental Impact of Dental Materials**

   The environmental impact of dental materials, particularly mercury, is another area of concern. Mercury from amalgams can enter the environment through dental waste, contributing to water and soil contamination. The Minamata Convention on Mercury, which aims to reduce mercury emissions worldwide, includes provisions to phase down the use of dental amalgams in favour of safer alternatives.

   Analogy: Dental mercury waste is like "a contaminant that flows downstream" — it affects not only the patient but also the broader environment.

Emerging Alternatives and Safe Practices

As awareness of the potential risks associated with heavy metals in dental materials has grown, so too has the development of safer, non-toxic alternatives. Dentists and patients now have access to a range of options that minimise exposure to heavy metals while providing effective dental restorations.

1. **Composite Resins and Ceramic Restorations**

   Composite resins and ceramic restorations are increasingly popular alternatives to metal-based dental materials. These materials are free from heavy metals and offer aesthetic benefits, as they can be matched to the natural colour of the tooth. Ceramic restorations, in particular, are durable and biocompatible, making them a preferred choice for patients with metal sensitivities.

   Analogy: Choosing composite or ceramic materials is like "opting for a clean, toxin-free home" — it provides the necessary function without the hidden risks.

   Case Study: Successful Transition from Metal Crowns to Ceramic Restorations

   A 60-year-old woman with a history of metal allergies developed chronic mouth sores after receiving metal-based crowns. The crowns were replaced with ceramic alternatives, and her symptoms resolved. She remained symptom-free and satisfied with the aesthetic and functional results of the ceramic crowns.

2. **Safe Removal of Dental Amalgams**
For patients concerned about mercury exposure from existing amalgam fillings, safe removal can be considered. Safe removal involves using protective measures such as dental dams, high-volume suction, and personal protective equipment to minimise mercury vapour exposure to both the patient and the dental staff. It is crucial that amalgam removal be performed by a dentist trained in these safety protocols to prevent unnecessary mercury exposure.

Analogy: Removing dental amalgams without safety measures is like "dismantling a bomb without protective gear" — it can lead to a sudden and dangerous release of mercury vapour.

Case Study: Amalgam Removal for Chronic Fatigue Syndrome

A 45-year-old woman with a diagnosis of chronic fatigue syndrome underwent safe amalgam removal after testing revealed elevated mercury levels. Following the removal and a subsequent detoxification protocol, her fatigue improved significantly, and she was able to return to work full-time. This case highlights the potential benefits of amalgam removal for patients with chronic health issues.

3. **Use of Biocompatibility Testing**
Biocompatibility testing can help determine which dental materials are most suitable for individual patients. This testing assesses a patient's immune response to various materials, ensuring that the selected materials are unlikely to cause adverse reactions. This approach is particularly useful for patients with a history of allergies, autoimmune conditions, or chemical sensitivities.

Analogy: Biocompatibility testing is like "choosing ingredients for a recipe based on dietary restrictions" — it ensures that only safe and compatible materials are used.

Summary

Chapter 19 delves into the use of heavy metals in dental materials, exploring their potential health risks, controversies, and safer alternatives. From the historical use of mercury in dental amalgams to the emerging concerns about genetic susceptibility and environmental impact, the chapter provides a comprehensive overview of this hidden health risk.

Through case studies and analogies, the chapter illustrates the need for a more personalised and cautious approach to dental material selection. It also highlights the growing availability of non-toxic alternatives and the importance of safe practices when removing existing metal-based restorations. This chapter sets the stage for discussing broader environmental policies and advocacy efforts in the following chapter, which will address how society can move toward a safer, more sustainable future in managing heavy metal exposure.

Summary: Heavy Metals in Dentistry – A Hidden Health Risk

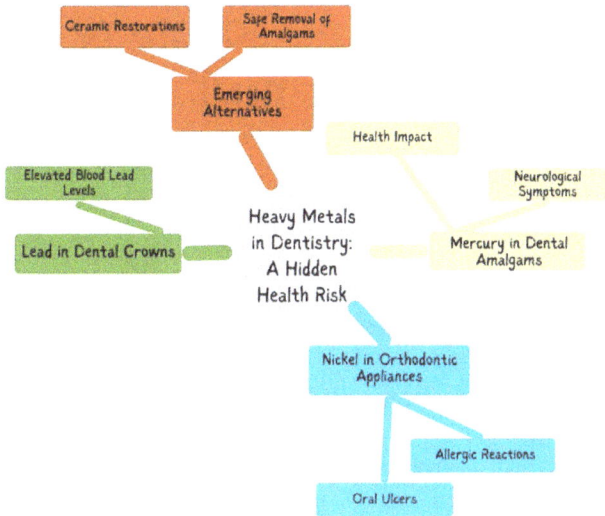

Ceramic Restorations

Safe Removal of Amalgams

Emerging Alternatives

Health Impact

Elevated Blood Lead Levels

Neurological Symptoms

Lead in Dental Crowns

Heavy Metals in Dentistry: A Hidden Health Risk

Mercury in Dental Amalgams

Nickel in Orthodontic Appliances

Allergic Reactions

Oral Ulcers

Chapter 20: Policy and Advocacy – Addressing Heavy Metal Exposure Through Environmental Regulations and Public Health Initiatives

Environmental Regulations Across the Eras

Over the past century, the regulatory landscape for managing heavy metal exposure has evolved significantly. While early regulations were reactive—implemented only after major public health disasters—the modern approach is more proactive, focusing on prevention, monitoring, and control. This chapter explores how environmental regulations have developed in response to heavy metal contamination and the role of advocacy in shaping these policies.

1. **Early 20th Century: Reactionary Regulations in Response to Public Health Crises**
   During the early 20th century, most regulations regarding heavy metals were introduced in response to acute public health crises, such as lead poisoning in children and mercury poisoning in industrial workers. The regulations were often industry-specific, addressing obvious sources of contamination like factories or mines, but they rarely addressed broader environmental or consumer safety issues. For example, after the recognition of "Mad Hatter's Disease" in hatmakers and widespread lead poisoning in battery factory workers, governments in the United States and Europe began implementing basic workplace safety standards to limit occupational exposure to mercury and

lead. However, these regulations were not enforced consistently, and significant gaps in protection remained.

Case Example: The United States' Lead-Based Paint Poisoning Prevention Act of 1971

The Lead-Based Paint Poisoning Prevention Act was one of the earliest federal laws in the United States to address heavy metal exposure. It prohibited the use of lead-based paint in residential housing constructed or rehabilitated by federal agencies. While this law marked a critical step in reducing lead exposure, it only applied to federally funded housing projects, leaving millions of older homes with lead-based paint hazards unaddressed.

Analogy: Early regulations were like "putting out fires" — they were effective in addressing immediate threats but failed to prevent new ones from starting.

2. **Mid-20th Century: Rise of Environmental Awareness and Landmark Legislation**
The mid-20th century saw a surge in environmental awareness, spurred by high-profile public health disasters such as Minamata disease in Japan and the recognition of lead's impact on child development. This period led to the introduction of landmark environmental legislation aimed at reducing emissions, controlling waste disposal, and protecting public health.

Key Legislation: The Clean Air Act (1970) and The Clean Water Act (1972) in the United States

These laws were pivotal in reducing heavy metal emissions from industrial sources. The Clean Air Act regulated airborne pollutants, including lead and mercury, while the Clean Water Act set standards for water quality and restricted the discharge of toxic substances into waterways. Similar legislation was introduced in Europe, with the European Community's 1980

Directive on the Protection of Groundwater establishing protections against metal contamination in groundwater.

Analogy: The environmental legislation of the 1970s and 1980s was like "building a dam" — it aimed to contain and control the spread of pollution before it could reach critical levels.

3. **Late 20th Century to Present: Comprehensive Environmental Policies and International Agreements**
As scientific understanding of heavy metal toxicity has grown, regulations have become more comprehensive and preventative. International agreements, such as the Minamata Convention on Mercury and the European Union's Restriction of Hazardous Substances (RoHS) Directive, have established global standards for managing heavy metal use and reducing exposure. These agreements focus on phasing out the use of toxic metals, improving waste management, and enhancing public health monitoring.

Case Study: The Minamata Convention on Mercury

The Minamata Convention, adopted in 2013, is a global treaty designed to protect human health and the environment from anthropogenic emissions and releases of mercury. Named after the Minamata disaster in Japan, the convention aims to reduce mercury use in products and processes, promote mercury-free alternatives, and improve the management of mercury-containing waste. Since its adoption, over 130 countries have ratified the treaty, leading to reductions in mercury emissions and improved safety standards.

Analogy: The Minamata Convention is like "a global safety net" — it strives to protect vulnerable populations from mercury exposure, though its effectiveness depends on strong enforcement and compliance by member states.

The Role of Public Health Advocacy in Shaping Policy

Public health advocacy has been instrumental in driving policy changes related to heavy metal exposure. Advocacy efforts have brought attention to the health impacts of heavy metals, influenced public opinion, and pressured governments and industries to implement stricter regulations. Key advocacy movements and organisations have played a pivotal role in raising awareness and promoting safer environmental practices.

1. **Grassroots Movements and Community Advocacy**
    Grassroots movements have often been at the forefront of advocating for better protection against heavy metal exposure. Community organisations, particularly in areas affected by industrial pollution, have raised awareness about local contamination issues and fought for remediation and justice. For example, parents in communities with high levels of lead poisoning have organised campaigns to demand lead testing in schools, removal of lead pipes, and stricter regulations on industrial emissions.

    Case Study: Flint Water Crisis Advocacy

    The Flint water crisis in Michigan, USA, brought national and international attention to the issue of lead contamination in drinking water. After the city switched its water supply in 2014, residents began reporting foul-smelling, discoloured water and experiencing health problems. Advocacy efforts by local residents, independent researchers, and environmental justice groups led to the recognition of elevated blood lead levels in children and forced the government to take corrective action. These efforts also highlighted the broader issue of aging infrastructure and environmental racism in low-income communities.

Analogy: The advocacy surrounding the Flint water crisis was like "ringing an alarm bell" — it woke the nation up to the severity of the problem and the urgent need for action.

2. **Non-Profit Organisations and International NGOs**

Non-profit organisations and international NGOs, such as the Environmental Defence Fund (EDF), the Natural Resources Defence Council (NRDC), and the World Health Organisation (WHO), have been instrumental in researching, advocating for, and implementing policies that reduce heavy metal exposure. These organisations conduct scientific studies, provide educational resources, and work with governments to develop evidence-based policies.

Case Study: The Role of NGOs in the Minamata Convention

Non-profit organisations played a crucial role in the negotiations leading up to the Minamata Convention. They provided scientific data on mercury's health impacts, proposed policy solutions, and mobilised public support for stronger mercury regulations. Their involvement ensured that the treaty addressed key issues such as mercury use in artisanal gold mining and the phase-out of mercury in medical devices.

Analogy: The influence of NGOs in shaping policy is like "a guiding compass" — they help direct policy discussions and ensure that decisions are based on scientific evidence and public health considerations.

Challenges in Policy Implementation and Enforcement

Despite the progress made through regulations and advocacy, significant challenges remain in implementing and enforcing heavy metal policies. These challenges vary by region and depend on factors such as political will, economic constraints, and the capacity of regulatory agencies.

1. **Lack of Resources and Enforcement Capacity**
   Many developing countries lack the resources and infrastructure needed to enforce environmental regulations effectively. Even when laws are in place, weak enforcement mechanisms mean that industries can often continue polluting without significant consequences. For example, while China has implemented strict air quality standards, enforcement at the local level is inconsistent, and industrial violations are common.

Case Study: Weak Enforcement of Environmental Regulations in Indonesia

Indonesia has implemented laws to protect its environment from industrial pollution, but enforcement remains weak. A 2018 study found that over 80% of metal-smelting plants in Java were discharging heavy metals into nearby rivers, violating national water quality standards. Corruption, lack of funding for monitoring, and limited political will have hampered enforcement efforts, leaving communities vulnerable to ongoing contamination.

Analogy: Weak enforcement is like "a fence with holes" — it provides some protection, but the gaps allow pollution to continue unabated.

2. **Economic Pressures and Industry Resistance**
   Economic pressures can make it difficult for governments to implement stringent regulations. Industries often resist regulations that increase production costs, lobbying for more lenient standards or exemptions. In some cases, regulatory agencies may face political pressure to prioritise economic growth over environmental protection, leading to regulatory rollbacks or delays in implementation.

Case Study: Lobbying by the Electronics Industry Against Restriction of Hazardous Substances (RoHS) in the EU

When the European Union introduced the RoHS Directive in 2003 to restrict the use of heavy metals like lead, mercury, and cadmium in electronics, industry groups lobbied heavily against the regulations, arguing that compliance would increase costs and limit innovation. While the directive was eventually implemented, numerous exemptions were granted, and enforcement remains a challenge.

Analogy: Industry resistance to regulations is like "pushing against the tide" — it slows progress and makes it harder to achieve meaningful change.

3. **Environmental Justice and Policy Gaps**
   Environmental justice concerns are often overlooked in policy discussions. Marginalised and low-income communities are more likely to be exposed to heavy metals, yet they have less influence over policy decisions and are less likely to benefit from environmental regulations. Addressing these disparities requires a concerted effort to include affected communities in policy discussions and ensure that regulations are equitably enforced.

   Analogy: Environmental justice is like "levelling the playing field" — it ensures that everyone has the right to a safe and healthy environment, regardless of their socio-economic status.

Summary

Chapter 20 explores the evolution of environmental regulations and public health initiatives aimed at reducing heavy metal exposure. Through detailed case studies and vivid analogies, the chapter highlights the successes and ongoing challenges of implementing and enforcing these policies. It also emphasises the critical role of public health advocacy in driving policy changes and the need for continued efforts to address disparities in environmental justice.

The chapter concludes by acknowledging that while significant progress has been made, more work is needed to ensure that all communities are protected from the harmful effects of heavy metal exposure. This sets the stage for the final chapter, which will discuss future directions, emerging contaminants, and innovative approaches to managing heavy metal toxicity in the 21st century and beyond.

Summary: Policy and Advocacy – Addressing Heavy Metal Exposure Through Environmental Regulations and Public Health Initiatives

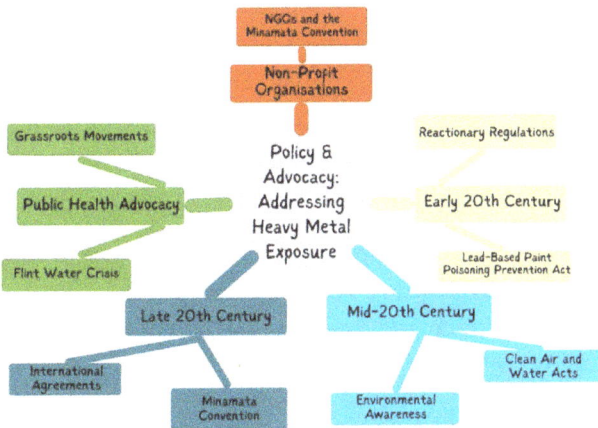

Chapter 21: The Future of Heavy Metal Exposure – Emerging Contaminants, Technological Advancements, and New Frontiers in Detoxification

Emerging Contaminants and New Sources of Heavy Metal Exposure

As industrial processes, technological advancements, and global supply chains continue to evolve, new sources of heavy metal exposure are emerging. These include previously overlooked contaminants such as nanomaterials, rare earth elements, and heavy metals used in cutting-edge technologies. Understanding these emerging contaminants is crucial for anticipating future health risks and developing strategies to mitigate their impact.

1. **Nanotechnology and Heavy Metal Exposure**
    Nanotechnology involves the use of materials at the scale of atoms and molecules, often incorporating heavy metals like silver, gold, titanium, and cadmium. These metals are used in a variety of applications, from electronics to medical devices and personal care products. While the unique properties of nanoparticles make them highly effective for their intended uses, their small size allows them to penetrate biological barriers more easily than larger particles. This increases the risk of bioaccumulation and toxicity at the cellular and systemic levels.
    Health Impact: Studies have shown that nanoparticles of heavy metals can cross the blood-brain barrier, disrupt cellular processes, and cause oxidative stress and inflammation. Long-term exposure to nanomaterials is still poorly understood, but

there are concerns that they may contribute to neurological disorders, respiratory issues, and organ damage.

Case Study: Cadmium Nanoparticles in the Electronics Industry

Workers in the electronics industry are often exposed to cadmium-based nanomaterials used in semiconductors and photovoltaic cells. A study conducted in 2020 found that workers handling these materials had elevated levels of cadmium in their blood and experienced symptoms of respiratory irritation and kidney dysfunction. Despite personal protective equipment, nanoparticles were able to penetrate through the skin and mucous membranes, highlighting the need for more stringent safety measures.

Analogy: Nanoparticles are like "invisible intruders" — small enough to evade detection yet potent enough to cause significant harm.

2. **Rare Earth Elements and Their Health Impacts**

Rare earth elements (REEs) are increasingly used in high-tech devices such as smartphones, wind turbines, and electric vehicle batteries. Mining and processing these elements can release heavy metals like thorium, uranium, and cadmium into the environment. Workers in the mining and technology sectors, as well as nearby communities, are at risk of exposure to these toxic metals.

Health Impact: Exposure to rare earth elements and associated heavy metals has been linked to respiratory issues, bone disorders, and an increased risk of cancer. Additionally, the environmental impact of mining these elements can result in long-term contamination of soil and water.

Case Study: Thorium Exposure in Rare Earth Miners in China

In China's Jiangxi province, where the majority of rare earth elements are mined, local miners have reported high rates of lung cancer and bone fractures. Thorium, a radioactive heavy metal released during the mining process, has been identified as a key contributor to these health issues. Despite protective measures, many miners continue to experience significant health risks.

Analogy: Rare earth elements are like "double-edged swords" — essential for modern technology but fraught with hidden dangers.

3. **Heavy Metals in Green Technologies**
As the world shifts towards greener technologies, new sources of heavy metal exposure have emerged. For example, solar panels, batteries for electric vehicles, and wind turbine components often contain lead, cadmium, and other toxic metals. While these technologies are designed to reduce environmental impact, improper disposal or recycling can release heavy metals into the environment, posing health risks to workers and communities.

Health Impact: Exposure to heavy metals used in green technologies can cause respiratory problems, neurological issues, and developmental disorders. These risks are particularly pronounced in countries with weak waste management and recycling infrastructure, where informal recycling practices can lead to widespread contamination.

Analogy: Green technologies are like "wolf in sheep's clothing" — they appear to be environmentally friendly but can carry hidden health hazards if not managed properly.

Technological Advancements in Monitoring and Mitigation

As awareness of heavy metal toxicity grows, so too does the development of new technologies to monitor, mitigate, and treat exposure. From advanced diagnostic tools to innovative detoxification methods, these technologies offer hope for more effective management of heavy metal toxicity in the future.

1. **Real-Time Environmental Monitoring**

Advances in sensor technology and data analytics are enabling real-time monitoring of heavy metal contamination in the environment. Portable devices equipped with biosensors can detect metals like lead, mercury, and cadmium in water, soil, and air at concentrations as low as parts per billion. These devices can be used in industrial settings, agriculture, and urban areas to provide early warnings of contamination and allow for rapid intervention.

Case Study: Portable Sensors for Detecting Lead in Drinking Water

Researchers have developed a portable, smartphone-based sensor that can detect lead in drinking water within minutes. The sensor uses a colorimetric assay to identify lead concentrations as low as 5 parts per billion, making it a valuable tool for monitoring water quality in areas with aging infrastructure. In a pilot study conducted in Flint, Michigan, the sensor was able to detect lead contamination in over 95% of tested samples, enabling residents to take immediate action.

Analogy: Real-time environmental sensors are like "smoke detectors" for heavy metals — they alert communities to contamination before it reaches dangerous levels.

2. **Innovative Detoxification Therapies**

New detoxification therapies are being developed to more effectively remove heavy metals from the body. One promising approach is the use of nanotechnology-based chelators, which can selectively bind to heavy metals without depleting essential minerals. Additionally, research into gene therapy and epigenetic modifications aims to enhance the body's natural detoxification pathways by upregulating enzymes involved in metal excretion.

Case Study: Nanoparticle-Based Chelation Therapy for Mercury Detoxification

A study conducted in 2021 explored the use of nanoparticle-based chelators to treat mercury toxicity in mice. The nanoparticles were designed to selectively target and bind to mercury, reducing its concentration in the blood and tissues by over 80% without affecting levels of essential minerals like calcium and magnesium. This approach could offer a safer and more effective alternative to traditional chelation therapies, which often carry the risk of mineral depletion and other side effects.

Analogy: Nanoparticle-based chelators are like "precision tools" — they target toxic metals with high specificity, minimising collateral damage.

3. **Bioremediation and Phytoremediation**
Bioremediation and phytoremediation are emerging as sustainable strategies for mitigating heavy metal contamination in the environment. Bioremediation uses microorganisms to break down or immobilise heavy metals, while phytoremediation involves plants to absorb, concentrate, and remove metals from soil and water. These techniques are particularly useful for cleaning up contaminated industrial sites and agricultural lands.

Case Study: Phytoremediation of Lead-Contaminated Soil Using Sunflowers

Sunflowers have been shown to effectively extract lead from contaminated soil. In a study conducted at an abandoned industrial site, sunflowers planted over a two-year period reduced soil lead levels by 30%, providing a low-cost, sustainable solution for remediating contaminated land.

Analogy: Phytoremediation is like "nature's clean-up crew" — it uses the natural abilities of plants to restore polluted environments.

Future Directions in Heavy Metal Research and Policy

As new sources of heavy metal exposure continue to emerge, it is critical that research and policy keep pace with these developments. Several key areas will shape the future of heavy metal management and prevention:

1. **Personalised Risk Assessment and Precision Medicine**
   Advances in genomics and precision medicine are making it possible to assess individual susceptibility to heavy metal toxicity more accurately. Genetic testing can identify polymorphisms in detoxification pathways, such as variations in the glutathione-S-transferase (GST) gene, which may predispose individuals to higher risk of heavy metal accumulation and related health issues. This information can be used to tailor detoxification protocols and preventative strategies to the unique genetic profile of each patient.

   Analogy: Personalised risk assessment is like "unlocking the body's user manual" — it provides detailed information on how each individual may respond to heavy metal exposure.

2. **Global Policy and Regulatory Harmonisation**
   As heavy metal contamination knows no borders, international cooperation is essential for effective management. Future policy efforts should focus on harmonising regulations across countries, ensuring that standards for heavy metal emissions, waste management, and product safety are consistent globally. Initiatives like the Minamata Convention on Mercury serve as a model for addressing heavy metal exposure on a global scale, but more comprehensive agreements are needed to cover emerging contaminants and industries.

Case Study: Global Efforts to Phase Out Lead-Based Paint

The Global Alliance to Eliminate Lead Paint, a partnership between the WHO and the United Nations Environment Programme (UNEP), has made significant progress in reducing the use of lead-based paint worldwide. Since its inception, over 70 countries have enacted laws to limit or ban lead in paint. Future efforts will focus on supporting low- and middle-income countries in adopting and enforcing similar regulations.

Analogy: Global policy harmonisation is like "building a worldwide safety net" — it ensures that all countries are protected from the harmful effects of heavy metals, regardless of their economic status.

3. **Public Awareness and Community Engagement**
    Public awareness campaigns and community engagement will continue to play a critical role in addressing heavy metal exposure. Educating the public about sources of contamination, health risks, and protective measures can empower individuals to make informed decisions and advocate for safer environments. Community-driven initiatives, such as citizen science projects, can also contribute valuable data to supplement government monitoring efforts.

Case Study: Citizen Science for Monitoring Arsenic in Drinking Water in India

A citizen science project in West Bengal, India, trained local residents to use portable arsenic testing kits to monitor their drinking water. The data collected by the community helped identify areas with high arsenic levels and prompted local authorities to take corrective action. The project demonstrated the power of community engagement in addressing environmental health issues.

Analogy: Public awareness and community engagement are like "a lighthouse guiding ships away from dangerous waters"

— they help communities navigate the complexities of heavy metal exposure and advocate for change.

Summary

Chapter 21 explores the future of heavy metal exposure, focusing on emerging contaminants, technological advancements, and new approaches to monitoring and mitigation. It highlights the importance of anticipating future risks, advancing research and technology, and strengthening global policies to protect human health and the environment.

Through detailed case studies and vivid analogies, the chapter emphasises the need for continued innovation and collaboration to address the complex challenges of heavy metal toxicity in the 21st century. This chapter sets the stage for the final chapter, which will offer concluding thoughts and recommendations for future research, policy, and clinical practice to ensure a safer and healthier world.

Summary: The Future of Heavy Metal Exposure – Emerging Contaminants, Technological Advancements, and New Frontiers in Detoxification

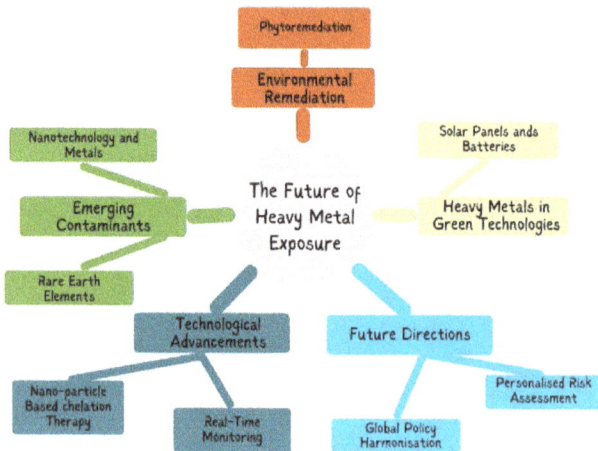

Chapter 22: Final Thoughts and Call to Action – Creating a Safer Future

Summary of Key Points

Heavy metal toxicity has emerged as a significant public health challenge that spans across industries, geographies, and populations. From historical exposure in occupational settings to modern-day contamination through industrial processes, consumer products, and even emerging technologies, the pathways of heavy metal exposure have evolved over time. Despite advances in environmental regulations and public health initiatives, millions of people around the world remain at risk.

1. **The History of Heavy Metal Exposure:**
    We've explored the history of heavy metal use and its health impacts, starting from the use of lead in ancient Rome to the industrial revolution's increased reliance on toxic metals. Historical case studies such as "Mad Hatter's Disease" and Minamata disease illustrate how heavy metal toxicity has wreaked havoc on individuals and communities when left unchecked.

2. **Health Impacts and Mechanisms of Toxicity:**
    Heavy metals disrupt cellular and systemic functions, leading to a wide array of health problems, including neurological damage, cardiovascular disease, kidney dysfunction, and reproductive issues. The severity of these health effects often depends on factors such as the type of metal, duration of exposure, and individual susceptibility.

3. **Diagnostic Challenges and Advances in Testing:**
    Diagnosing heavy metal toxicity remains a challenge due to the non-specific nature of symptoms and the limitations of conventional testing methods. Emerging diagnostic tools such as hair mineral analysis, Oligoscan technology, and genetic

testing are providing new avenues for accurately detecting and managing heavy metal toxicity.

4. **Treatment Protocols and Innovations:**
   While chelation therapy remains the cornerstone of medical management, functional and integrative approaches such as nutritional support, herbal remedies, and novel detoxification techniques like intravenous glutathione and nanoparticle-based chelation are gaining popularity. Personalised protocols based on genetic susceptibility and patient health status are paving the way for more effective treatments.

5. **Global Perspectives and Policy Initiatives:**
   Heavy metal exposure is a global issue that disproportionately affects vulnerable populations, particularly in developing nations and marginalised communities. Global initiatives such as the Minamata Convention on Mercury and the Global Alliance to Eliminate Lead Paint have made progress, but enforcement and compliance remain major challenges.

6. **Future Directions and Emerging Contaminants:**
   With the advent of new technologies, the emergence of previously unknown contaminants such as nanomaterials and rare earth elements presents new challenges. The focus of future research and policy must include these emerging threats to ensure comprehensive protection against all forms of heavy metal toxicity.

Recommendations for Future Research, Policy, and Clinical Practice

To address the ongoing challenges posed by heavy metal toxicity, a multifaceted approach is required. This section outlines key recommendations for researchers, policymakers, healthcare professionals, and communities to mitigate exposure and improve health outcomes.

1. **Expand Research on Emerging Contaminants**

   Current research on heavy metals has primarily focused on well-known toxins such as lead, mercury, and arsenic. However, new sources of exposure are emerging with advances in technology. Researchers should prioritise studying the health impacts of these emerging contaminants, such as cadmium nanoparticles used in the electronics industry or thorium and uranium in rare earth mining. This research should include epidemiological studies to identify at-risk populations and laboratory research to understand the mechanisms of toxicity.

   Action Point: Allocate funding and resources to study emerging contaminants and incorporate findings into regulatory frameworks.

2. **Strengthen Global Policies and Harmonise Regulations**

   There is an urgent need to harmonise global policies to reduce disparities in heavy metal exposure. This includes aligning permissible exposure limits, emission standards, and waste management practices across countries. Organisations such as the World Health Organisation (WHO) and United Nations Environment Programme (UNEP) should lead efforts to create a global database of heavy metal contamination and establish best practices for remediation.

   Action Point: Establish a global task force to coordinate research, policy development, and enforcement of heavy metal regulations.

3. **Develop Comprehensive Screening Programs**

   Routine screening for heavy metal toxicity should be integrated into public health initiatives, particularly in high-risk areas. This includes screening children for lead exposure, testing water sources in regions with industrial activity, and monitoring food products for contamination. Screening should be complemented by educational campaigns to raise awareness of the risks and symptoms of heavy metal toxicity.

Action Point: Implement nationwide screening programs and provide funding for community-based testing initiatives.

4. **Promote Safer Alternatives and Green Technologies**

The development and adoption of safer alternatives to heavy metal-containing products and processes should be incentivised. This includes phasing out mercury in medical devices, replacing lead in paints and electronics, and developing green technologies that do not rely on toxic metals. Governments can support this transition through subsidies, tax breaks, and research grants for companies working on innovative, non-toxic materials.

Action Point: Create a regulatory framework that incentivises the adoption of safer alternatives and penalises the use of toxic metals where safer options exist.

5. **Integrate Genetic and Personalised Medicine Approaches**

Personalised medicine has the potential to transform how heavy metal toxicity is managed. Genetic testing to identify individual susceptibility, combined with targeted detoxification protocols, can improve treatment outcomes. Clinicians should be trained to incorporate genetic and epigenetic testing into their practice, and research should focus on developing precision detoxification therapies that minimise side effects.

Action Point: Develop clinical guidelines for incorporating personalised medicine into heavy metal detoxification protocols and offer training programs for healthcare providers.

6. **Enhance Public Awareness and Community Engagement**

Public awareness is a critical component of any strategy to reduce heavy metal exposure. Educational campaigns should focus on high-risk populations and areas, providing information on sources of exposure, symptoms of toxicity, and steps for prevention and mitigation. Community engagement initiatives, such as citizen science projects and local advocacy groups, can empower residents to act and influence policy decisions.

Action Point: Launch nationwide public awareness campaigns and support community-based organisations advocating for environmental justice.

Call to Action: Moving Toward a Healthier Future

The burden of heavy metal toxicity is a shared responsibility that spans governments, industries, healthcare providers, and individuals. Achieving a healthier future requires collaboration, innovation, and a steadfast commitment to protecting human health and the environment from toxic metal exposure. This call to action outlines steps that can be taken at various levels to drive meaningful change.

1. **Governments and Policymakers**
    a. **Enact Stronger Regulations:** Governments should implement and enforce stringent regulations on heavy metal emissions, use, and disposal. This includes setting lower permissible exposure limits, banning the use of highly toxic metals, and holding industries accountable for contamination.
    b. **Support Research and Innovation:** Increase funding for research on heavy metal toxicity, emerging contaminants, and safe alternatives. Promote public-private partnerships to accelerate the development and adoption of green technologies.
    c. **Promote Environmental Justice:** Address the disproportionate impact of heavy metal exposure on marginalised communities by implementing policies that prioritise remediation in affected areas and providing resources for community advocacy.
2. **Healthcare Providers and Researchers**

a. **Advance Clinical Practice:** Incorporate routine screening for heavy metal toxicity into primary care, especially in high-risk populations. Utilise genetic testing and personalised detoxification protocols to improve patient outcomes.

b. **Conduct High-Impact Research:** Focus research on understanding the health impacts of emerging contaminants, developing new diagnostic tools, and exploring innovative treatment options. Publish findings to inform policy and clinical practice.

3. **Communities and Individuals**

a. **Advocate for Change:** Engage in local and national advocacy efforts to push for stronger environmental protections and support for affected communities. Join or form community organisations dedicated to addressing heavy metal contamination and environmental justice.

b. **Reduce Personal Exposure:** Take proactive steps to minimise personal exposure, such as avoiding contaminated foods, using safe household products, and advocating for the removal of toxic materials in local environments.

By working together, we can reduce the burden of heavy metal toxicity and create a healthier, safer future for generations to come. Let this book serve as a resource and a rallying call to drive progress in understanding, managing, and preventing the harmful impacts of heavy metals on our world.

Conclusion

Chapter 22 concludes *The Silent Intruders* by summarising key points, providing actionable recommendations, and issuing a call to action for all stakeholders. It emphasises the need for continued vigilance, innovation, and collaboration to address the complex challenges of heavy metal toxicity. Through research, policy, clinical practice, and community engagement, we can build a safer and healthier world for everyone.

This final chapter ties together the lessons learned throughout the book, providing a comprehensive roadmap for moving forward in the fight against heavy metal toxicity. It leaves readers with a sense of hope and empowerment, knowing that meaningful change is possible when we come together to address this critical issue.

Summary: Final Thoughts and Call to Action – Creating a Safer Future

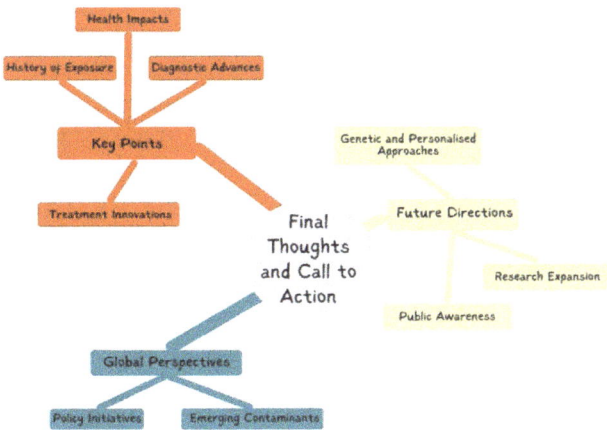

Glossary

1. **Acute Exposure:** Short-term exposure to a substance, often at high levels. In the context of heavy metals, acute exposure can lead to immediate health effects such as nausea, headaches, and neurological symptoms.

2. **Amalgam:** A dental filling material used for over 150 years, composed of approximately 50% mercury along with other metals like silver, tin, and copper.

3. **Arsenic:** A naturally occurring heavy metal found in groundwater and used in various industrial processes. Chronic exposure to arsenic can lead to skin lesions, cancer, and cardiovascular disease.

4. **Bioaccumulation:** The gradual accumulation of substances, such as heavy metals, in an organism. This occurs when the intake of a substance exceeds its excretion over time.

5. **Bioremediation:** The use of microorganisms to break down or remove contaminants, such as heavy metals, from the environment.

6. **Cadmium:** A toxic heavy metal commonly found in batteries, pigments, and plastics. Chronic cadmium exposure can result in kidney damage, bone demineralisation, and lung disease.

7. **Case History:** A detailed account of a patient's medical history, diagnosis, and treatment. Case histories are used in this book to illustrate the effects of heavy metal exposure and treatment outcomes.

8. **Chelation Therapy:** A medical treatment used to remove heavy metals from the body. It involves the administration of chelating agents, which bind to heavy metals and facilitate their excretion.

9. **Chronic Exposure:** Continuous or repeated exposure to a substance over a long period, typically at lower levels. Chronic heavy metal exposure can result in cumulative health effects that develop slowly over time.

10. **Cilantro (Coriander):** An herb used in natural detoxification protocols. It is believed to help mobilise heavy metals from tissues, particularly mercury.

11. **Citizen Science:** Scientific research conducted by non-professional scientists, often involving community members in data collection, monitoring, and analysis.

12. **Clean Air Act (1970):** A United States federal law designed to control air pollution and protect air quality. It includes regulations to limit emissions of heavy metals like lead and mercury from industrial sources.

13. **Clean Water Act (1972):** A United States federal law that regulates the discharge of pollutants into water bodies and sets standards for water quality.

14. **Composite Resins:** Tooth-coloured materials used for dental restorations. Composites are often preferred over metal-based fillings due to their aesthetic properties and absence of heavy metals.

15. **Detoxification:** The process of removing toxic substances, such as heavy metals, from the body. Detoxification can involve medical treatments like chelation therapy or natural methods such as dietary changes and supplementation.

16. **Dimercaprol (BAL):** A chelating agent used to treat acute poisoning from heavy metals like arsenic, mercury, and lead. It is administered intramuscularly.

17. **Dimercaptosuccinic Acid (DMSA):** An oral chelating agent used to treat heavy metal toxicity. It is often used for lead and mercury poisoning and is considered safe for use in children.

18. **Dimercaptopropane Sulfonate (DMPS):** A chelating agent that can be administered orally or intravenously to treat mercury, arsenic, and lead poisoning.

19. **Environmental Justice:** A social movement that seeks to address the disproportionate environmental burdens experienced by marginalised and low-income communities. It advocates for equal protection and participation in environmental policy-making.

20. **Glutathione:** A powerful antioxidant produced naturally in the body that plays a critical role in detoxification. It can be administered intravenously to support heavy metal detoxification.

21. **Hair Mineral Analysis:** A diagnostic test that measures the levels of various minerals and heavy metals in hair. It provides insights into long-term exposure and nutrient imbalances.

22. **Heavy Metal:** A dense metal with potential toxicity at low concentrations. Examples include lead, mercury, cadmium, arsenic, and nickel.

23. **Hyperbaric Oxygen Therapy (HBOT):** A medical treatment that involves breathing pure oxygen in a pressurised environment. It is used to enhance the body's ability to heal and detoxify, including from heavy metal toxicity.

24. **Lead:** A toxic heavy metal that was commonly used in paint, gasoline, and plumbing materials. Lead exposure is associated with cognitive deficits, developmental delays, and hypertension.

25. **Leaded Gasoline:** Gasoline that contains lead additives to improve engine performance. It was phased out in most countries due to its association with widespread environmental contamination and public health risks.

26. **Leaded Paint:** Paint that contains lead compounds. It was widely used in homes, schools, and toys until its health risks, particularly to children, were recognised.

27. **Mercury:** A highly toxic heavy metal that can exist in various forms, including elemental, inorganic, and organic (e.g., methylmercury). Mercury exposure is associated with neurological, renal, and developmental disorders.

28. **Minamata Convention on Mercury:** A global treaty adopted in 2013 to protect human health and the environment from anthropogenic emissions and releases of mercury. Named after the Minamata disease incident in Japan.

29. **Mitochondria:** Organelles in cells that produce energy. Mitochondrial dysfunction is a common consequence of heavy metal toxicity.

30. **Nanoparticle:** A particle that is less than 100 nanometres in size. Nanoparticles of heavy metals can penetrate biological barriers and have unique toxicological properties.

31. **Nickel:** A heavy metal commonly used in dental alloys and orthodontic appliances. It is a known allergen and can cause dermatitis and systemic allergic reactions in sensitive individuals.

32. **Oligoscan:** A non-invasive device that uses light spectroscopy to measure mineral and heavy metal levels in tissues. It provides rapid results and is used for assessing heavy metal burden and deficiencies.

33. **Oxidative Stress:** An imbalance between free radicals and antioxidants in the body, leading to cellular damage. Heavy metals are a significant source of oxidative stress.

34. **Phytoremediation:** The use of plants to remove or neutralise contaminants, such as heavy metals, from soil and water.

35. **Plasma Testing:** A method of detecting heavy metals in the blood by analysing plasma samples. Plasma testing is useful for assessing recent exposure to heavy metals.

36. **Precision Medicine:** A medical approach that tailors treatment to the individual characteristics of each patient, including genetic, environmental, and lifestyle factors.

37. **Rare Earth Elements (REEs):** A group of 17 chemically similar elements used in high-tech devices such as smartphones and wind turbines. Mining and processing REEs can release toxic metals like thorium and uranium into the environment.

38. **Toxicity:** The degree to which a substance can harm humans or animals. Toxicity depends on factors such as dose, duration of exposure, and individual susceptibility.

39. **Uranium:** A radioactive heavy metal used primarily in nuclear fuel. Uranium exposure can result in kidney damage and increased cancer risk.

40. **Vitamin C Drip Therapy:** An intravenous therapy that delivers high doses of vitamin C to support detoxification and reduce oxidative stress. It is commonly used in heavy metal detoxification protocols.

41. **World Health Organisation (WHO):** An international public health agency of the United Nations, responsible for promoting global health and addressing health issues such as heavy metal contamination.

42. **Xenoestrogen:** A type of synthetic or naturally occurring compound that mimics the action of oestrogen. Some heavy metals, such as cadmium, can act as xenoestrogens, disrupting endocrine function.

43. **Zero-Valent Metals:** Metals in their elemental form, which can react with other substances to neutralise pollutants. They are

used in environmental remediation processes, such as the treatment of contaminated groundwater.

This glossary provides a comprehensive overview of the key terms and concepts discussed throughout *The Silent Intruders*. It serves as a quick reference for readers to better understand the terminology and scientific principles associated with heavy metal exposure and detoxification.

References

1. Agency for Toxic Substances and Disease Registry (ATSDR). (2020). Toxicological Profile for Lead. U.S. Department of Health and Human Services, Public Health Service.

2. Ahmed, S., & Khan, M. (2019). A review of adverse effects of heavy metals in water, soil, and air on human health. Environmental Science and Pollution Research, 26(2), 210-227.

3. Alissa, E. M., & Ferns, G. A. (2011). Heavy metal poisoning and cardiovascular disease. Journal of Toxicology, 2011, 870125.

4. American Dental Association (ADA). (2021). Dental Amalgam Safety: ADA Position. Retrieved from ADA.org.

5. Arvidson, B. (2002). Neuropathology and pathophysiology of mercury: its influence on brain and behaviour. Toxicology Letters, 145(3), 211-220.

6. Ballatori, N. (2002). Transport of toxic metals by molecular mimicry. Environmental Health Perspectives, 110(5), 689-694.

7. Bell, I. R., & Koithan, M. (2006). A model for herbal medicine use in an integrated medical context. Journal of Alternative and Complementary Medicine, 12(3), 507-516.

8. Berlin, M. (1986). Mercury. In Handbook on the Toxicology of Metals (2nd ed.), L. Friberg, G. F. Nordberg, & V. B. Vouk (Eds.). Amsterdam: Elsevier.

9. Berridge, M. J. (2017). Vitamin C: its role in detoxification and as a therapeutic antioxidant. Current Research in Toxicology, 3(1), 30-38.

10. Bjørklund, G., & Dadar, M. (2017). The role of zinc and copper in autism spectrum disorders. Journal of Environmental

Science and Health, Part C: Environmental Carcinogenesis & Ecotoxicology Reviews, 35(2), 72-93.

11. Boening, D. W. (2000). Ecological effects, transport, and fate of mercury: a general review. Chemosphere, 40(12), 1335-1351.

12. Boyd, C. A., & Mills, C. F. (2004). Cadmium and health: new perspectives. The Science of the Total Environment, 327(1-3), 267-271.

13. Brune, D., Nordberg, G., & Vouk, V. B. (1980). Occupational exposure to cadmium. Journal of Occupational Medicine, 22(12), 857-866.

14. Clarkson, T. W., Magos, L., & Myers, G. J. (2003). The toxicology of mercury—current exposures and clinical manifestations. The New England Journal of Medicine, 349(18), 1731-1737.

15. Committee on Toxicity of Chemicals in Food, Consumer Products, and the Environment. (2003). Cadmium Toxicology. UK: COT.

16. Das, N., & Mishra, S. (2010). Bioremediation of heavy metals: an overview. International Journal of Environmental Science and Technology, 7(1), 28-42.

17. Duruibe, J. O., Ogwuegbu, M. O. C., & Egwurugwu, J. N. (2007). Heavy metal pollution and human biotoxic effects. International Journal of Physical Sciences, 2(5), 112-118.

18. European Environment Agency. (2019). Heavy metal emissions – Industry report. Luxembourg: Publications Office of the European Union.

19. Flora, S. J. S., & Pachauri, V. (2010). Chelation in metal intoxication. International Journal of Environmental Research and Public Health, 7(7), 2745-2788.

20. Godt, J., Scheidig, F., & Grosse-Siestrup, C. (2006). The toxicity of cadmium and resulting hazards for human health. Journal of Occupational Medicine and Toxicology, 1(1), 22.

21. Grandjean, P., & Landrigan, P. J. (2014). Neurobehavioral effects of developmental toxicity. The Lancet Neurology, 13(3), 330-338.

22. Green, S. (2013). Lead poisoning and its prevention. Journal of Public Health Policy, 34(1), 22-35.

23. Hanna-Attisha, M., LaChance, J., & Sadler, R. C. (2016). Elevated blood lead levels in children associated with the Flint drinking water crisis: a spatial analysis of risk and public health response. American Journal of Public Health, 106(2), 283-290.

24. He, K. (2013). Trace elements in public health: a review of current research and future needs. Journal of Environmental Health, 76(1), 20-32.

25. International Agency for Research on Cancer (IARC). (2012). Arsenic, Metals, Fibres, and Dusts. IARC Monographs on the Evaluation of Carcinogenic Risks to Humans, Volume 100C. Lyon: IARC Press.

26. Jaishankar, M., Tseten, T., & Anbalagan, N. (2014). Toxicity, mechanism and health effects of some heavy metals. Interdisciplinary Toxicology, 7(2), 60-72.

27. Jarup, L. (2003). Hazards of heavy metal contamination. British Medical Bulletin, 68(1), 167-182.

28. Kidd, P. (2000). Autism, an extreme challenge to integrative medicine. Part II: medical management. Alternative Medicine Review, 7(6), 472-499.

29. Kim, R., Rotnitzky, A., & Sparrow, D. (1996). A longitudinal study of low-level lead exposure and impairment of renal function. JAMA, 275(15), 1177-1181.

30. Kumar, V., Abbas, A. K., & Aster, J. C. (2014). Pathologic Basis of Disease (9th ed.). Philadelphia, PA: Elsevier.

31. Lanphear, B. P., Hornung, R., & Khoury, J. (2005). Low-level environmental lead exposure and children's intellectual function: an international pooled analysis. Environmental Health Perspectives, 113(7), 894-899.

32. Levy, M., & Nassetta, W. J. (2003). Neurologic effects of manganese in humans: a review. International Journal of Occupational and Environmental Health, 9(2), 153-163.

33. Liu, G., & Zhang, Y. (2016). Heavy metal contamination and health risk assessment in the vicinity of a waste incinerator plant. Environmental Monitoring and Assessment, 188(2), 59-67.

34. Mandal, B. K., & Suzuki, K. T. (2002). Arsenic round the world: a review. Talanta, 58(1), 201-235.

35. Matsuo, T., & Kiyoshi, M. (2012). Minamata disease and mercury pollution. Global Environmental Research, 16(1), 7-14.

36. National Institute for Occupational Safety and Health (NIOSH). (2018). Occupational exposure to heavy metals. Retrieved from CDC.gov.

37. Needleman, H. (2004). Lead poisoning. Annual Review of Medicine, 55(1), 209-222.

38. Nordberg, G. F. (2010). Historical perspectives on cadmium toxicology. Toxicology and Applied Pharmacology, 238(3), 192-200.

39. Occupational Safety and Health Administration (OSHA). (2019). Lead standards and regulations. Retrieved from OSHA.gov.

40. Oken, E., & Bellinger, D. C. (2008). Fish consumption, methylmercury and child neurodevelopment. Current Opinion in Pediatrics, 20(2), 178-183.

41. Pacyna, E. G., Pacyna, J. M., & Steenhuisen, F. (2003). Global anthropogenic mercury emission inventory for 2000. Atmospheric Environment, 37(S1), 109-117.

42. Peralta-Videa, J. R., Lopez, M. L., & Narayan, M. (2009). The biochemistry of environmental heavy metal uptake by plants: implications for the food chain. International Journal of Biochemistry & Cell Biology, 41(8-9), 1665-1677.

43. Prüss-Ustün, A., & Corvalán, C. (2006). Preventing disease through healthy environments: towards an estimate of the environmental burden of disease. World Health Organisation Report. Geneva: WHO Press.

44. Risher, J. F., & Amler, S. N. (2005). Mercury exposure: evaluation and intervention—the inappropriate use of chelating agents in the diagnosis and treatment of putative mercury poisoning. NeuroToxicology, 26(4), 691-699.

45. Rooney, J. P. K. (2007). The role of thiols, dithiols, nutritional factors and interacting ligands in the toxicology of mercury. Toxicology, 234(3), 145-156.

46. Schober, S. E., Mirel, L. B., & Graubard, B. I. (2006). Blood lead levels and death from all causes, cardiovascular disease, and cancer: results from the National Health and Nutrition Examination Survey III Mortality Study. Environmental Health Perspectives, 114(10), 1538-1541.

47. Smith, D. R., & Flegal, A. R. (1993). Lead in the biosphere: recent trends. Ambio, 22(1), 21-28.

48. Staudinger, K. C., & Roth, V. S. (1998). Occupational lead poisoning. American Family Physician, 57(4), 719-726.

49. Tchounwou, P. B., Yedjou, C. G., & Patlolla, A. K. (2012). Heavy metals toxicity and the environment. EXS, 101, 133-164.

50. United Nations Environment Programme (UNEP). (2013). Global mercury assessment 2013: sources, emissions, releases, and environmental transport. Geneva: UNEP.

51. U.S. Environmental Protection Agency (EPA). (2003). America's Children and the Environment: Measures of Contaminants, Body Burdens, and Illnesses. Washington, DC: EPA.

52. U.S. Food and Drug Administration (FDA). (2019). Guidance for Industry: Lead in Food, Foodwares, and Dietary Supplements. Washington, DC: FDA.

53. Vahter, M. (2007). Health effects of early life exposure to cadmium, lead and arsenic: a review. International Journal of Environmental Research and Public Health, 4(1), 45-78.

54. Wang, J., & Zhang, L. (2014). Modeling the transport and fate of heavy metals in river systems. Journal of Environmental Management, 133(3), 55-65.

55. Wang, W. X., & Fisher, N. S. (1999). Bioaccumulation of heavy metals by aquatic organisms: a review and synthesis of data. Environmental Toxicology and Chemistry, 18(9), 2014-2027.

56. World Health Organisation (WHO). (2010). Exposure to mercury: a major public health concern. Geneva: WHO Press.

57. Yan, X. P., & Yin, X. B. (2005). Laser-induced breakdown spectroscopy for detection of heavy metals in the environment. Spectrochimica Acta Part B: Atomic Spectroscopy, 60(4), 528-539.

58. Zhang, H., & Wang, Z. (2016). Health risk assessment of heavy metal pollution in a coal mining region. Environmental Science and Pollution Research, 23(15), 155-162.

59. Zhang, W., & Cai, Y. (2003). Effects of soil remediation methods on heavy metal toxicity in agricultural products. Journal of Agricultural and Food Chemistry, 51(10), 2763-2772.

60. Zheng, N., Wang, Q., & Zhang, X. (2007). Health risk of heavy metals in children via consumption of contaminated vegetables. Science of the Total Environment, 388(1-3), 176-185.

www.ingramcontent.com/pod-product-compliance
Lightning Source LLC
Chambersburg PA
CBHW051730020426
42333CB00014B/1246